Contents

Contents

Contents

Section 1
INTRODUCTION AND BACKGROUND

"It is health that is real wealth and not pieces of gold and silver."

— Mahatma Gandhi

Introduction

Hi, my name is Zak and I will be your guide through the world of health and type 2 diabetes!

I am a Health Advisor - I deliver sessions for the NHS Diabetes Prevention Programme, run my own health education programme in London and Essex, and offer 1-1 health consultations.

In this book I will address topics such as nutrition, exercise, stress, sleep, inflammation, gut health, and much more, in order to give you a holistic view of your health, with tools to make changes.

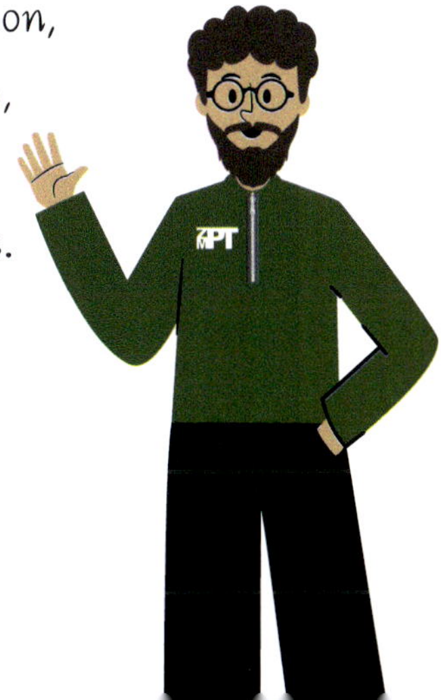

This is not just my guide to type 2 diabetes, it is my guide to good health. My hope is that anyone who wants to make a change to their health can use this book to do so.

My background

I have always worked in health and sport. As a child, I was a competitive swimmer, and I have been a swim coach since the age of 16. At 18, I became a personal trainer and began helping people exercise more and eat healthier.

I later attended university and studied Sport and Exercise Science, exploring topics such as sports nutrition, anatomy and physiology, strength and conditioning, biomechanics, and sport psychology. I particularly enjoyed studying the ways in which the brain and body connect.

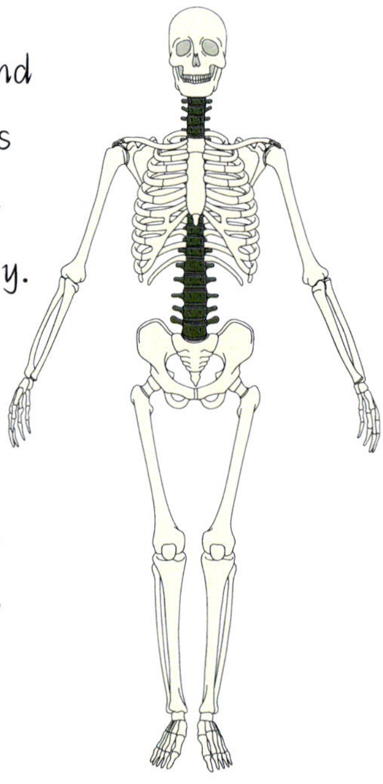

Now, my career is centred around helping people improve their health and there is nothing I find more gratifying. I truly hope you enjoy reading this book as much as I have enjoyed writing it!

Navigating your health

I like to compare the topic of health to a large, complex map, because there are many routes a person can take to improve their health, and the pursuit itself is a journey.

I also make this comparison because it can be easy to get lost, or led to believe that there is only one route to your destination, when in fact, there are many ways of improving your health, just as there are many paths that lead to the same location.

The purpose of this book is to help you understand the map, the various routes you can take, the subtle nuances of health, and the ways in which it all connects. Diabetes is simply the topic I am using to demonstrate this.

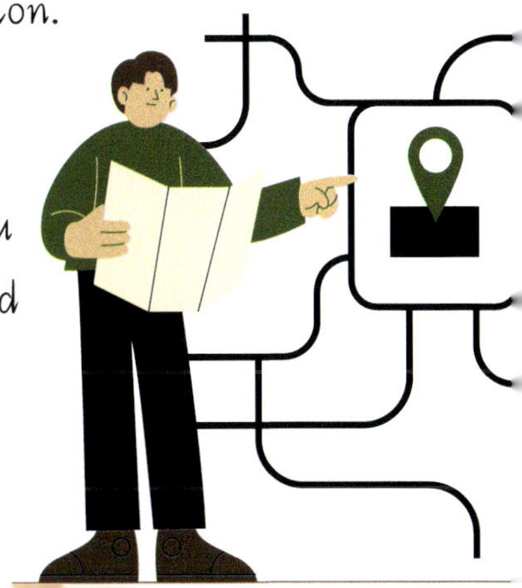

The history of health

The Greek physicians Hippocrates (460-370 BC) and Galen (129-210 AD) have influenced much of modern medicine.

Hippocrates is known as the 'Father of Medicine', who moved away from prayer and sacrifice to improve health; and towards diet, medicine, and exercise. 'The Hippocratic Oath' is attributed to Hippocrates and his involvement in medicine.

Galen began studying medicine at 16 and would teach the '7 Laws of Health'. These included: breathing fresh air, eating the correct foods, drinking the right beverages, getting enough sleep, having a daily bowel movement, controlling one's emotions, and exercising. This holistic view still carries weight today.

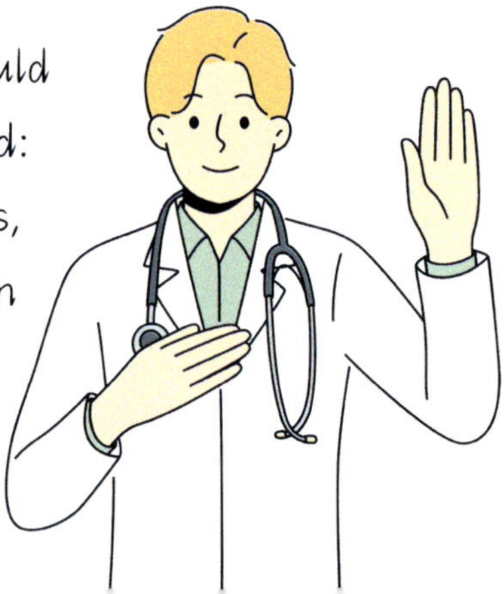

The history of diabetes

Type 2 diabetes has been studied for over 4000 years by various cultures and societies throughout history.

The full name for diabetes is 'Diabetes mellitus'. Diabetes is a Greek word to describe something 'being siphoned'. The word mellitus is a Latin word, meaning 'sweet'. The two words together refer to the fact that when your blood sugar is high, the excess sugar is siphoned out of your body through urine, making the urine sweet.

In fact, to test people for diabetes, physicians used to taste urine - if it was sweet, this was an indicator of diabetes. Fortunately, as of the last 100 years, we now know how to prevent and treat diabetes - type 1 and type 2.

Diabetes fact file

Currently, around 830 million people globally have diabetes - 90-95% of them have type 2 diabetes.

4.6 million people in the UK have type 2 diabetes.

An estimated 1.3 million people in the UK are diabetic and undiagnosed.

In 2021, globally, 1.6 million deaths were caused by diabetes related conditions.

Life expectancy of people with type 2 diabetes drops by an average of 10%.

Between 2016 and 2023, the number of young people (25 years and under) diagnosed with type 2 diabetes increased by 54%!

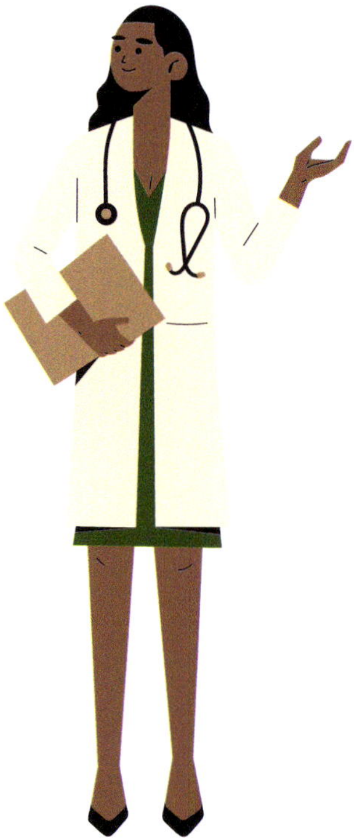

What is Type 2 Diabetes?

Type 2 diabetes is a chronic condition which indicates that the body is not regulating blood sugar correctly. As a result, a person with type 2 diabetes will likely have consistently high blood sugar levels, which can lead to severe health complications such as cardiovascular disease, amputations, and blindness (to name a few).

High blood sugar levels are often the result of insulin resistance, and a lack of insulin production - both of which will be explained further on page 10.

There are many factors which affect your risk of developing this condition, hence why this book goes into detail about so many different topics. It is therefore important to consider your health from a holistic point of view.

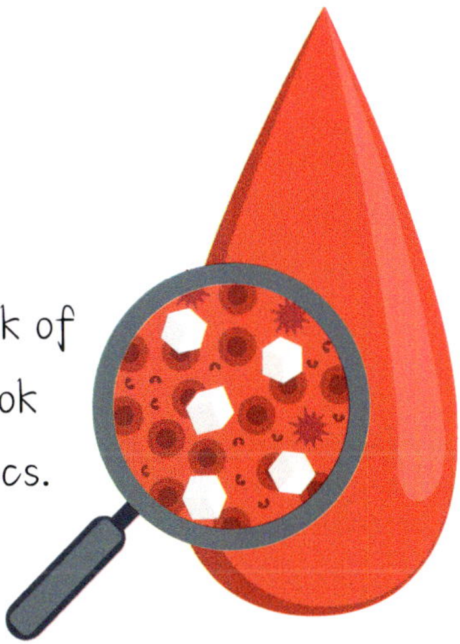

Blood glucose/sugar

Glucose is sugar in its simplest form. If your blood sugar is rising, this means the level of glucose in your blood is increasing. This is why we use the phrases 'blood glucose' and 'blood sugar', often interchangeably.

Glucose is the body's primary energy source!

It is a common misconception that blood sugar is ONLY affected by what you eat. In reality, your blood sugar will rise and fall throughout the day, for a variety of reasons, many of which we will explore throughout this book. The important thing to remember is that these changes are normal.

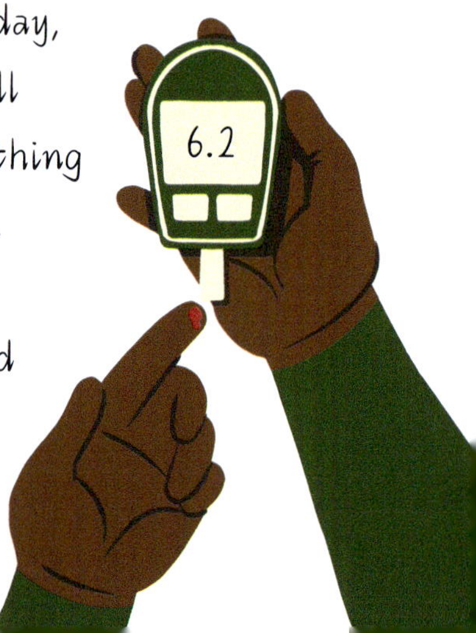

It only becomes a health concern if your blood sugar is consistently too high, because this affects how your body produces, and responds to insulin.

Insulin

Insulin is a hormone that is produced within the beta cells of the pancreas, and is released into the bloodstream when your blood sugar increases. Insulin allows the cells in your body (e.g. muscle cells, brain cells, liver cells) to feed off of the glucose in your blood.

The glucose is then converted to energy, which enables the cells to function. As the glucose is converted, your blood sugar levels will decrease. The time it takes for your blood sugar to fall depends on your level of insulin sensitivity.

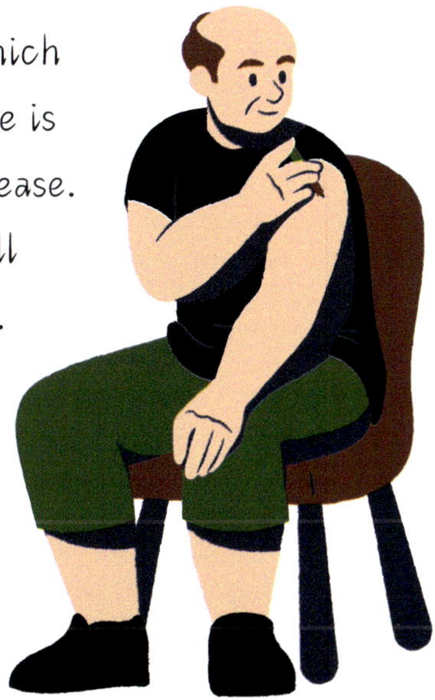

Insulin sensitivity refers to how well your body cells respond to insulin. If your cells are more insulin sensitive, your blood sugar should fall sooner when insulin levels rise.

Insulin resistance and production

If your blood sugar levels are consistently too high, the cells can become less sensitive to insulin - this is called insulin resistance. This is like your cells are getting fed up, going on strike, and ignoring the insulin.

Type 1 diabetics naturally produce very little insulin or none at all.

This means less glucose is being used as energy, and instead, stays in the blood.

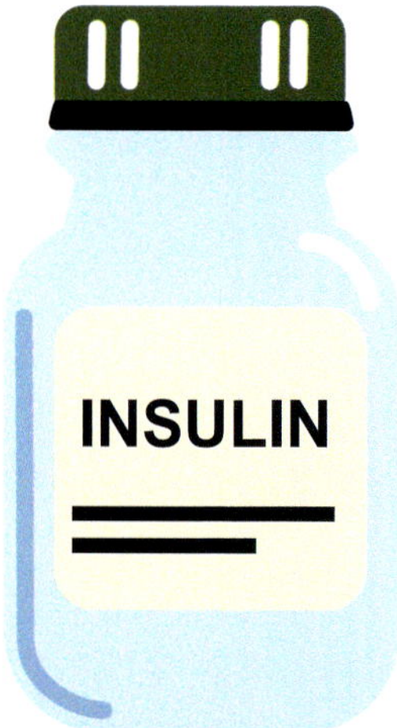

As well as becoming insulin resistant, people with type 2 diabetes also begin producing less insulin. This is because the beta cells, which produce insulin (page 9), become worn out.

Therefore, as a result of insulin resistance and reduced insulin production, your blood sugar levels are likely to get even higher over time.

HBA1C

Your HBA1C result is an indicator of how high or low your blood sugar has been, on average, for the past 3 months. It is also a measure of whether you are diabetic, pre-diabetic, or normal.

HBA1C is created when your blood sugar levels are too high, for too long, initiating a process called glycation.

Glycation occurs when glucose accumulates in the blood, and becomes very sticky, attaching itself to proteins in the body. HBA1C is created when glucose sticks to a protein called Haemoglobin, which transports oxygen around the body. If your HBA1C number is higher, it means that more glycation has occurred, because your blood sugar levels have been elevated.

HBA1C values

The table below outlines whether a person is in the normal, pre-diabetic, or diabetic range, depending on their HBA1C value. You can request an HBA1C test from your GP, or ask them for your result if you are unsure what it is.

It is possible to reduce this number by following the guidance in this book. However, not everyone experiences a reduction, and it can take longer than you might expect. Therefore, it is important to focus on the changes you make, not just the results.

Normal	Pre-diabetic	Diabetic
41 and below	42 to 47	48 and above

Measured in mmol/mol

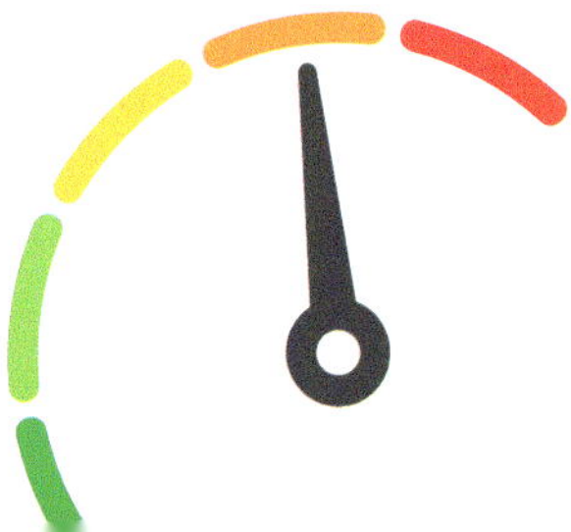

Symptoms

Below is a list of symptoms which are common for people with type 2 diabetes to develop. It is important that you do not ignore symptoms.

There are people who are pre-diabetic who get symptoms early, and there are diabetics who don't get any symptoms at all. In any case, it is important to get tested annually (at least).

Excessive thirst	Frequent urination
Fatigue and tiredness	Blurred vision
Recurrent thrush	Slow wound healing
Weight fluctations	Gingivitis

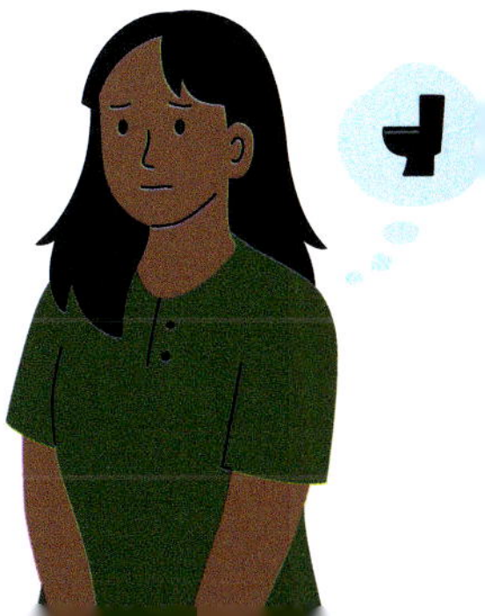

Complications

Glycation (mentioned on page 11) occurs when your blood sugar is consistently too high, and can have a catastrophic effect on your health. This is because glycation damages the nerves and cells around the entire body.

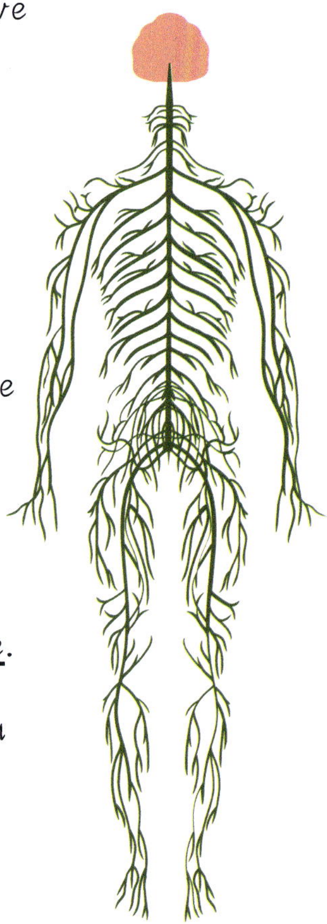

Imagine your body was a building. Your nerves would be the wiring, and your cells would be the bricks. In this analogy, glycation would cause the entire building to deteriorate, and this is what happens to the body when your blood sugar is consistently too high.

In short, continuously high blood sugar = damage.

Following the guidance in this book can help you control your blood sugar better and prevent the complications listed on the next page.

Complications

The table below highlights the potentially life threatening and life altering complications that are associated with type 2 diabetes.

It is not a guarantee that you will develop all or any of them, but the bottom line is that it can happen. I hope to help you avoid them!

Cardiovascular disease	Heart attacks
Kidney disease/failure	Strokes
Erectile dysfunction	Blindness
Gum disease	Nerve damage and amputations

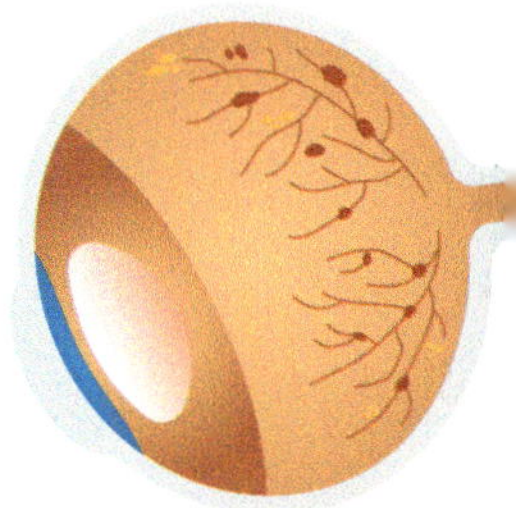

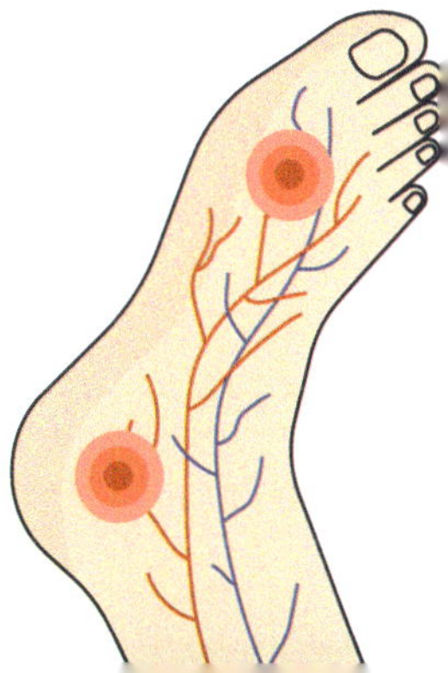

Overview of type 2 diabetes

Type 2 diabetes is a condition which indicates that the body is not regulating blood sugar as it should.

When your blood sugar is continuously and excessively high, your body cells may become insulin resistant, and your pancreas may also produce less insulin. The combined effect is that your blood sugar will become even less regulated.

Over time, high blood sugar levels can cause glycation, damaging nerves and cells around the entire body, leading to severe health complications. Fortunately, you can avoid and treat type 2 diabetes by focussing on lifestyle factors like those listed on the next page.

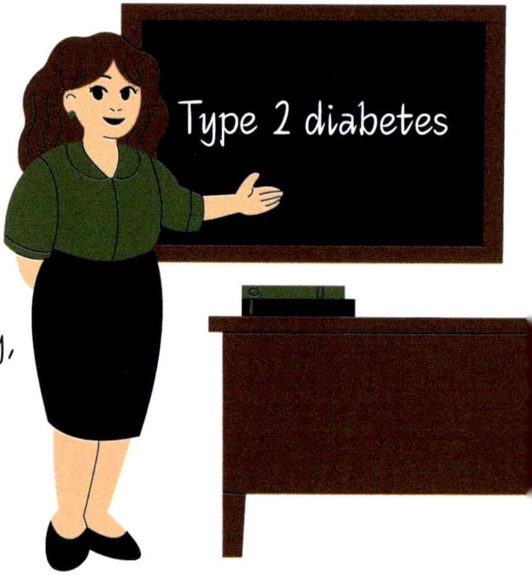

What causes type 2 diabetes?

Moving forward, the following factors can ALL affect the development of type 2 diabetes, directly and indirectly.

- Nutrition and hydration
- Physical activity
- Excess body fat
- Chronic stress
- Lack of sleep
- Alcohol
- Caffeine
- Nicotine
- Certain medications
- Chronic inflammation
- Oxidative stress
- Gut health issues
- Hormonal changes and fluctuations

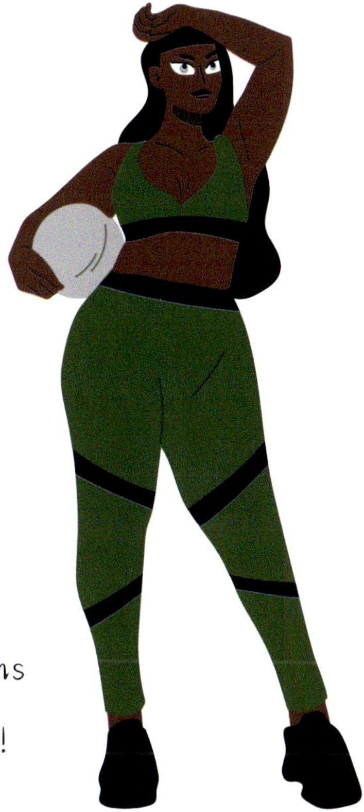

These are the topics we will explore further!

Risk factors

In addition to the lifestyle factors listed on the previous page, the following risk factors are important to consider, but are out of your control. Though it is important to be aware of these factors, remember to focus on those which are under your control.

- Age - the older you get, the higher your chances are of developing type 2 diabetes because bodily processes slow down.

- Genetics - if a parent or sibling has type 2 diabetes, you are 2-6 times more likely to develop it yourself.

- Ethnicity - you are 4 times more likely to develop type 2 diabetes if you are of South Asian, African, or Caribbean descent.

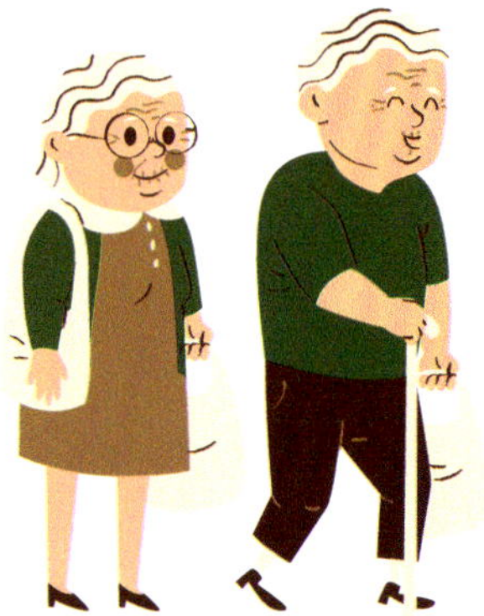

Additional risk factors for women

This is a list of risk factors which are specific to women:

- Gestational diabetes - a temporary form of diabetes which occurs during pregnancy, and increases the likelihood of developing type 2 diabetes later in life for both the mother and child.

- Polycystic ovary syndrome - this condition is often linked to increased insulin resistance and blood sugar levels, both of which increase the risk of type 2 diabetes.

- Peri-menopause and menopause - the hormonal changes and fluctuations that are associated with menopause can also cause an increase in insulin resistance and blood sugar, and therefore the risk of type 2 diabetes.

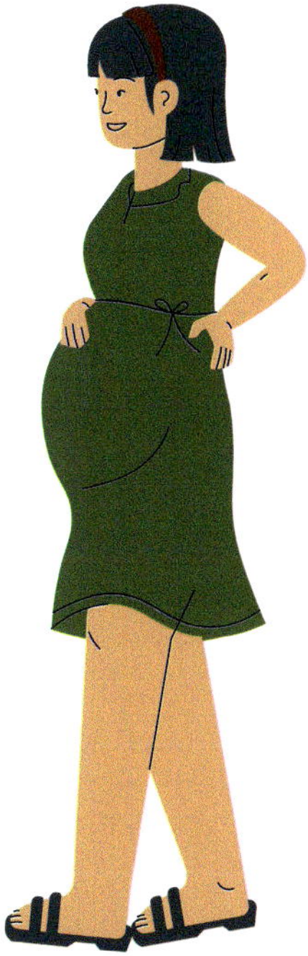

Making a change

As you will discover in the upcoming sections, many factors affect your health, and it can be difficult to know where to start. Fortunately, you don't need to make drastic changes to see improvements in your health.

You are more likely to find success by making small, incremental, and enjoyable adjustments. Otherwise, you risk making changes that are too big, or make you unhappy, and how long is that likely to last?

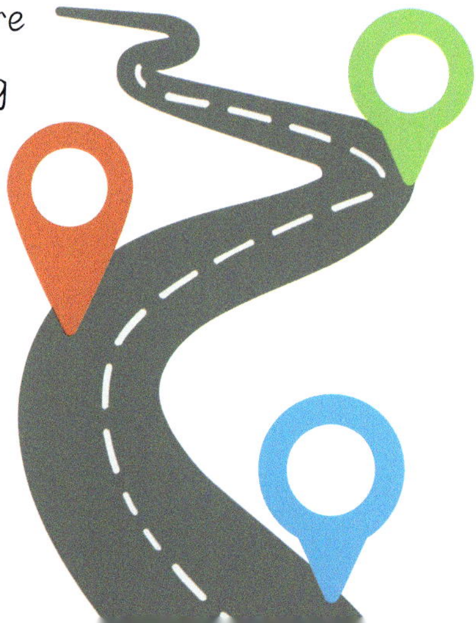

Hopefully, the information within this book will highlight alterations that you can see yourself making, but, don't attempt to tackle it all at once.

Making a change

On page 161, I have included a structure which you can use to create a plan for moving forward. For now, and as you read through the upcoming sections, I would encourage you to take some time and ask yourself the following questions, in order to establish your <u>aims</u> for the future.

- What do I hope to achieve by reading this book?
- What are my problem areas?
- What is in my control?
- What changes could I make today that I might enjoy?
- What changes have I made so far?

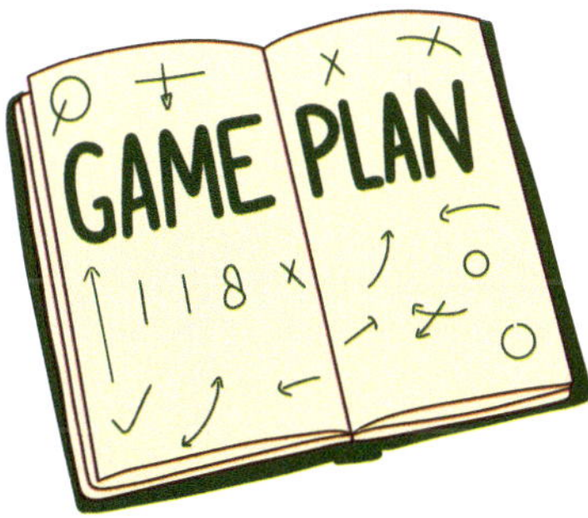

Reflection point 1

This is a list of suggestions based on the information from this section:

- Recognise the importance of blood glucose/sugar and insulin.
- Ask your GP for your HBA1C number if you don't know it, and get tested as frequently as you can.
- Seek out treatment if you start to notice any symptoms or complications, and warn others if they begin to experience them.
- Write down the factors which are affecting your risk of developing type 2 diabetes.
- Separate the factors which you can and cannot control.
- Ask yourself the questions on page 21 and establish your aims for moving forward.

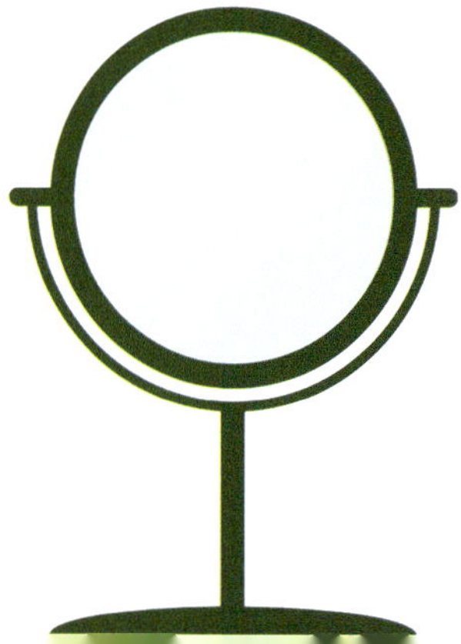

Section 2
NUTRITION AND EATING HABITS

"The doctor of the future will no longer treat the human frame with drugs, but rather will cure and prevent disease with nutrition."

— Thomas Edison

The history of nutrition

Human beings have been around for 5-6 million years, and up until 10,000 years ago, we were mainly hunter-gatherers. But by 2000 years ago, most people were farmers and relied on agriculture for their food, which we still rely on today. This was a relatively quick change in human history.

Grasslands became home to wheat, rye, barley, and rice; and animals like dogs, cattle, sheep, goats, pigs, and horses were domesticated. These changes helped us provide for a growing population that no longer had to travel vast distances to find food or water. However, as a result of cultivating select crops and livestock, the variety in our diet decreased, and this began to contribute to new diet-related illnesses. Later, food processing and overconsumption would create new issues.

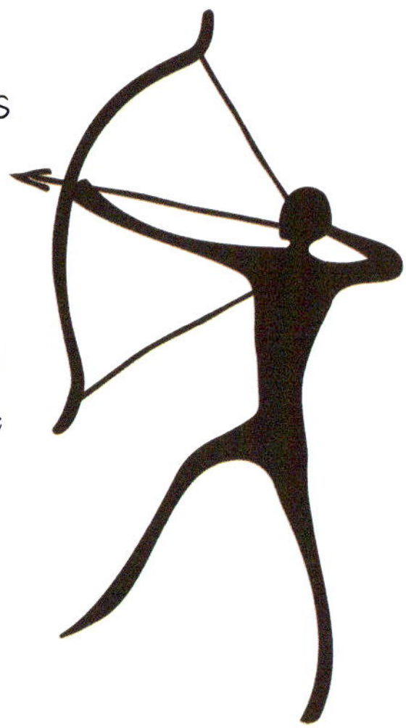

Nutrition

In this section, I will explain various aspects of nutrition and suggest methods for improving your own.

There is no need to make dramatic changes, nor would I expect anyone to cut anything completely from their diet, unless they want to. I also do not intend to demonise food. It is our relationship with food which makes it healthy or not.

When it comes to nutrition, I believe in balance and understanding. Food is a large part of our lives - socially, culturally, and biologically. However, if you understand how different foods affect your health, it can make you more aware of the decisions you make.

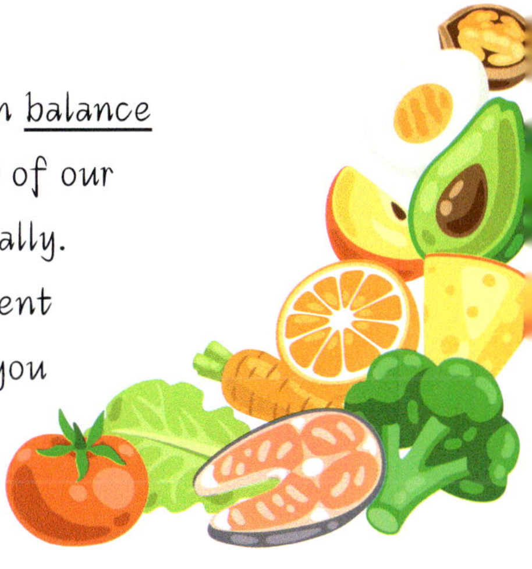

Carbohydrates

A carbohydrate is classed as any food that contains sugar and/or starch. This includes foods like biscuits, cakes, sweets, bread, rice, pasta, dairy products, fruit, vegetables, beans, pulses, lentils, grains, seeds, nuts, and more.

Starch and sugar are both digested by the body and converted into glucose, which is the body's primary energy source (page 8). The speed that the food is digested will affect how quickly the glucose enters your bloodstream, where your body can then use it for energy.

Some carbohydrates affect blood sugar more than others. This is due to the Glycemic Index.

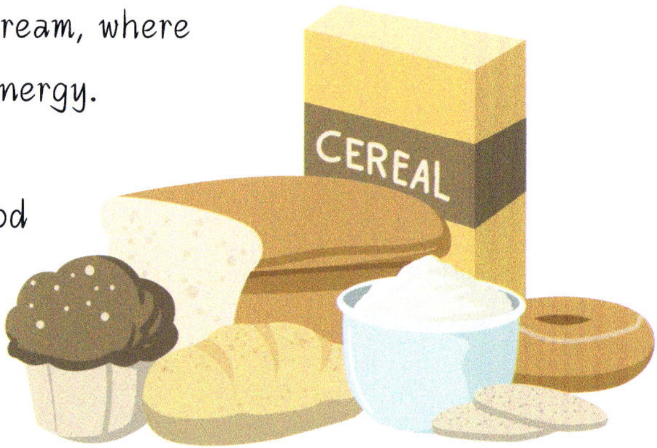

Glycemic Index

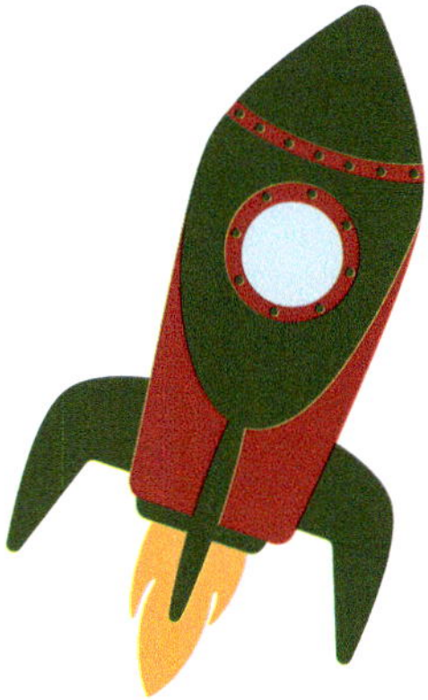

Glycemic Index (or GI) is a measure of how different foods affect blood sugar. Higher GI foods cause a larger rise in blood sugar, whereas lower GI foods cause a smaller rise in blood sugar.

The graph below demonstrates this difference. However, this is merely a representation, blood sugar doesn't always change exactly like this.

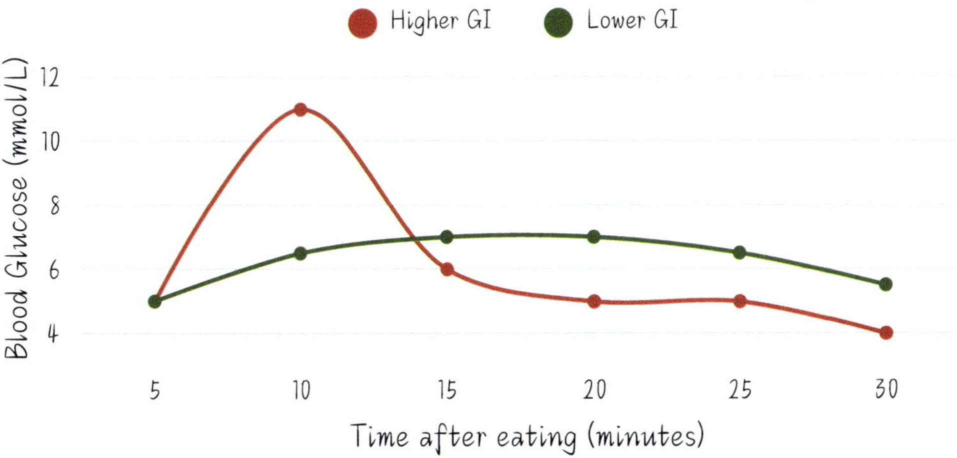

Blood sugar and energy

Most of your energy comes from the glucose/sugar inside of your blood. Higher GI foods can cause a larger rise in blood sugar, often followed by a crash. This may translate to a burst of energy, followed by a slump. This is because they are generally digested quicker, meaning glucose enters the bloodstream faster.

Lower GI foods, on the other hand, cause a smaller rise, and a slower fall. This is because they are digested slower, due to the presence of fat, fibre, and protein. Meaning lower GI foods can help you keep your blood sugar stable and prolong your energy levels.

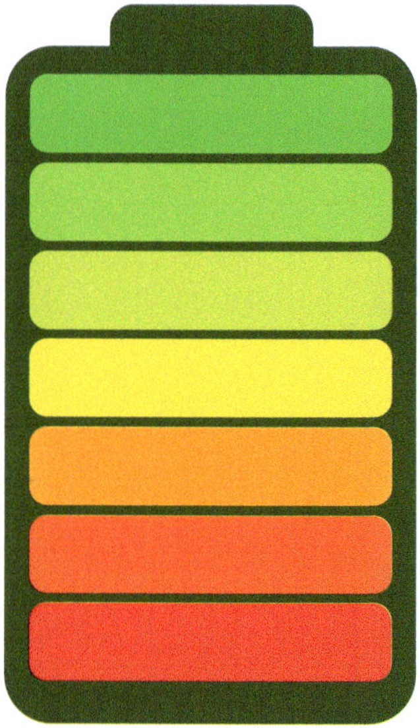

Use the next two pages to identify which foods in your diet are causing your blood sugar to rise more and less.

Lower GI examples

These are examples of lower GI foods.

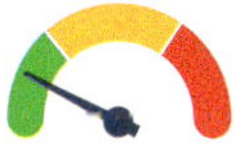

	Lower GI foods
Fruits	Berries, pomegranate, plums, citrus fruits, apples, pears, cherries, kiwi, apricots, prunes, and less ripe banana - (all unsweetened)
Vegetables, grains and legumes	Non-starchy vegetables, sweet potato, new potato, beans, chickpeas, lentils, peas, soy, quinoa, bulgar wheat, nuts, and seeds
Dairy and dairy alternatives	Milk, cheese, cream, cream cheese, yoghurt, almond milk, soy milk, and coconut milk - (all unsweetened)
Starchy foods	Brown, wild, and basmati rice, seeded wholemeal bread, sourdough bread, rye bread, wholemeal pasta, and wholegrain oats
Syrups and honey	Maple syrup, agave nectar, and raw/unrefined honey
Sugars	Coconut sugar and date sugar

Higher GI examples

These are examples of higher GI foods.

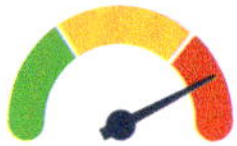

	Higher GI foods
Fruits	Pineapple, melon, grapes, and riper banana, canned fruit in syrups and juice, cooked fruit, and sweetened dried fruit
Vegetables, grains and legumes	White potatoes, parsnips, pumpkin, and vegetables, grains, and legumes which have been cooked and/or highly processed
Dairy and dairy alternatives	Dairy products with added sugar, rice milk, and oat milk
Starchy foods	White bread, white pasta, white rice, highly processed cereals, microwave rice, and instant oats
Syrups and honey	Glucose syrup, high fructose corn syrup, brown rice syrup, molasses, and refined/pasteurised honey
Sugars	White sugar, brown sugar, cane sugar, caster sugar, demerara, and jaggery

Adjusting the GI

Based on the information from the previous two pages, you can make food swaps in favour of those with a lower GI. However, that isn't the only thing you can do.

Foods that have a higher GI are not inherently bad, and don't need to be removed entirely from your diet. This is because you can adjust individual foods, meals, and snacks so that they don't impact your blood sugar quite as much.

There are several things you can change which should help you control your blood sugar. These include: the variety on the plate, the order and timing of how you eat the food, and the way the food is prepared. The next few pages contain a few suggestions, give them a try!

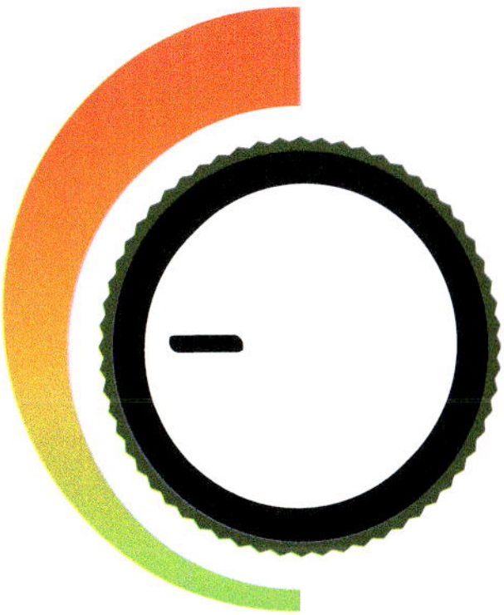

Fat, fibre, and protein

Fat, fibre, and protein all digest slower than carbohydrates. Therefore, eating these nutrients alongside carbohydrates can slow down the rate that the starch and sugar are converted into glucose, meaning blood sugar doesn't rise as high or as fast. This is why many of the lower GI examples contain larger quantities of fat, fibre, and protein, in comparison to the higher GI examples.

You can actually add fat, fibre, and protein to a meal or snack, and thereby, reduce the impact it has on your blood sugar. An extra serving of vegetables or chicken can make a difference. You could add fibrous foods like those on page 35, healthy fats from page 42, and proteins from page 45.

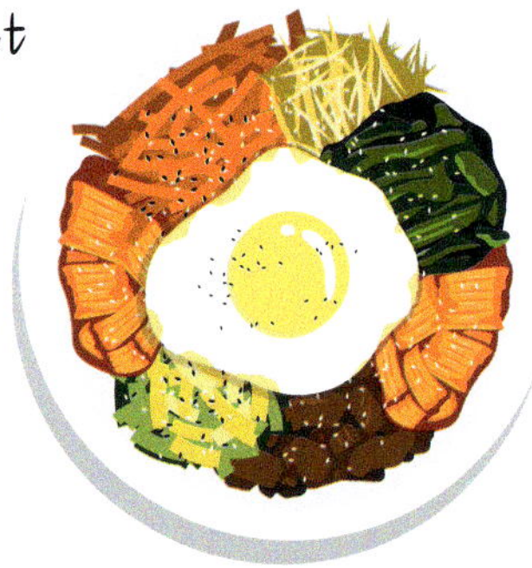

Order and timing

Adding fat, fibre, and protein to your plate helps to slow the rate of digestion. To slow digestion even further, you can start your meal or snack by eating the fat, fibre, and protein first.

For instance, if you were eating fish, chips, and vegetables; you could eat the fish and vegetables first, and the chips last. This should reduce the effect that the chips have on your blood sugar.

Alternatively, you could save snacks and treats for after you finish your meal, rather than eating them on an empty stomach. For example, instead of eating a chocolate bar now, you could save it for dessert. This can then be applied to all of the higher GI foods.

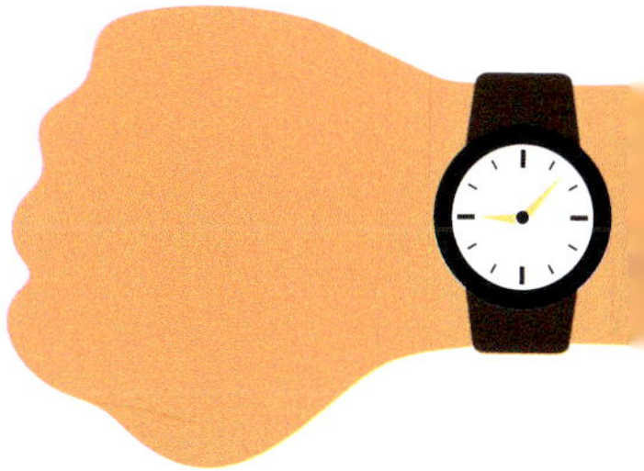

You can also adjust how you prepare certain carbohydrates. For instance, when making pasta, rice, or potatoes, you could allow them to cool down. This will cause some of the starch to become resistant starch, which has a lower glycemic index. You could then reheat it or eat it cold and it will still affect blood sugar less!

Make sure to cool rice quickly, only reheat it once, and reheat it to a high temperature!

You could also cook them so that they are 'al-dente', this will make these carbohydrates slower to digest, which will prevent your blood sugar from rising as high or as fast. Finally, you can also rinse the starch from rice before it is cooked, and from pasta after it is cooked, and this too can reduce the impact on your blood sugar because there is less starch to convert into glucose.

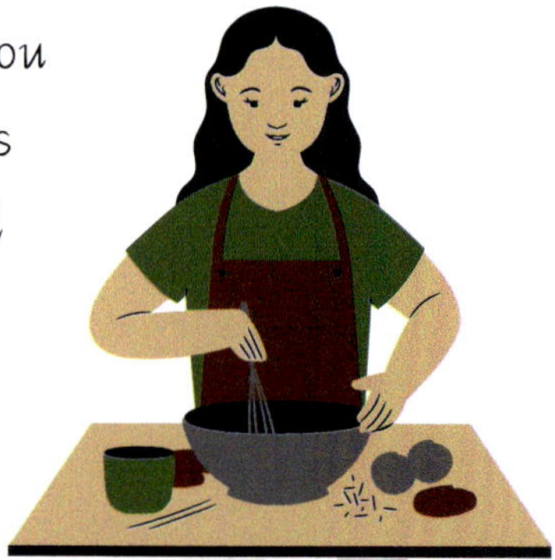

Fibre

The two types of fibre are soluble and insoluble. Soluble fibre dissolves in water to form a gel-like substance, which aids in slowing down digestion, reducing blood sugar spikes, reducing cholesterol levels (page 37), and improving gut health (145).

Insoluble fibre does not dissolve in water, instead it remains largely intact, preventing constipation and aiding in the elimination of waste products.

Most fibrous foods contain insoluble and soluble fibre. Therefore, I recommend gradually adding a wide variety of fibrous foods to your diet, attempting to eat at least 30g per day.

People who eat more fibre are at lower risk of developing type 2 diabetes, cardiovascular disease, diverticulitis, haemorrhoids, and bowel cancer!

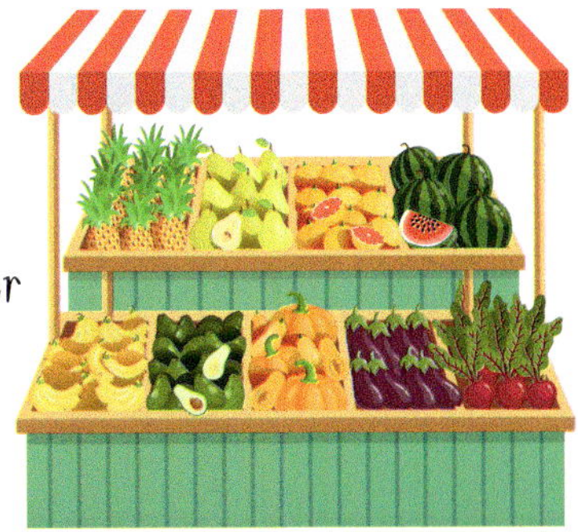

Foods that contain fibre

You can use this table to add fibre to your diet, make food swaps, and find new snack ideas. However, there are plenty of other fibrous foods to choose from.

Wholegrain pasta, bread, rice, oats	Bulgar wheat, barley, popcorn, quinoa
Apples, oranges, pears, berries, cherries, plums	Beans, lentils, peas, chickpeas, edamame
Bananas, grapes, melon, pineapple, dates, prunes	Sweet potato, new potato, potato skins
Peppers, mushrooms, courgettes, avocado	Nuts, seeds

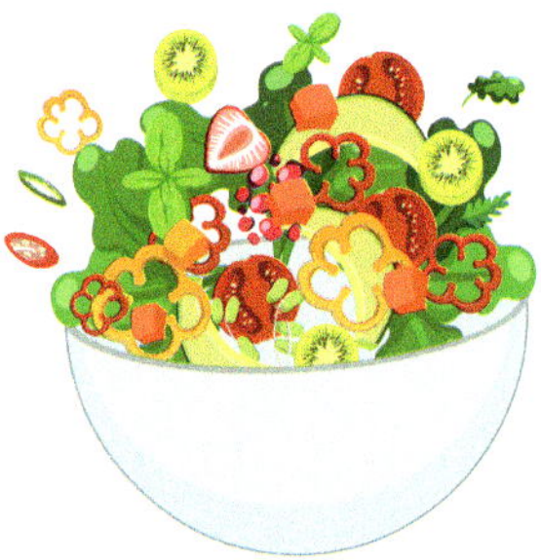

Fat

Fats are a confusing and polarising topic. We often assume that fat is bad, but that isn't always the case.

Including more fats in your diet can help you to improve your blood sugar, as mentioned on page 31. However, there are multiple types of fat which can affect your health in different ways. This is, in part, due to the effect they have on your cholesterol.

Understanding the different types of fat, the connection between fat and cholesterol, and the types of fat which will benefit you most and least, can help you reduce your risk of developing cardiovascular disease and type 2 diabetes.

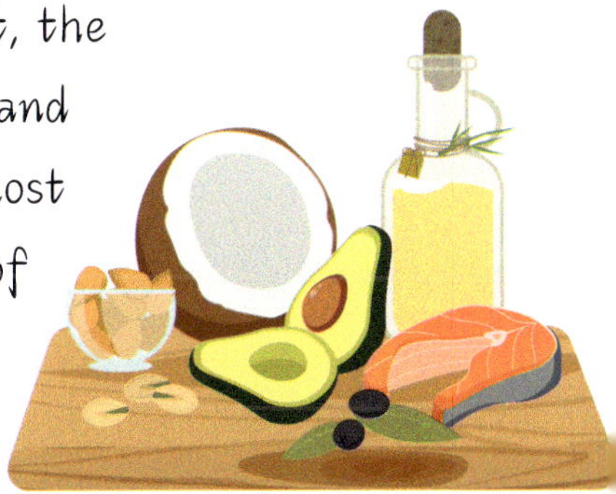

Fats and cholesterol

Fats and cholesterol are types of lipids, and neither are inherently bad. They are simply compounds which have different jobs to complete around the body. For example; fats are a source of energy, which can help the body absorb vitamins, produce hormones, and allow cells to function correctly. Cholesterol is a waxy substance that also aids in hormone production, as well as digestion, and maintaining the immune system.

The difference is that cholesterol cannot be burnt to produce energy, it can only be transported around the body and recycled. Therefore, cholesterol binds to proteins and fats to create lipoproteins, this is the vessel that carries cholesterol through the blood.

Like a cargo ship!

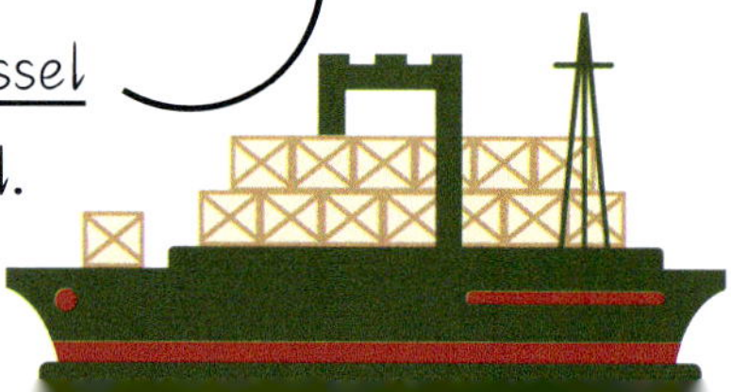

Lipoproteins

There are multiple types of lipoprotein, most people know of 'Low Density Lipoproteins' and 'High Density Lipoproteins', or LDLs and HDLs.

LDLs and HDLs both carry cholesterol through the body. However, when LDLs oxidise, they can cause an inflammatory response within the blood vessels, causing plaque to build up. This build up can lead to blockages, and cardiovascular disease, heart attacks, and strokes. Therefore, it is not cholesterol that is bad, but how it is transported around the body.

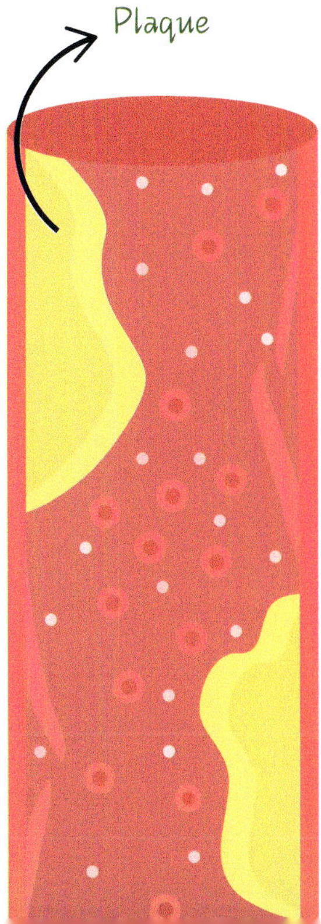

HDLs, on the other hand, transport cholesterol through the blood without causing that plaque to build up. HDLs can even help to "clean" your blood vessels of plaque. Therefore, it is healthier to have more HDLs than LDLs in your blood.

Unsaturated fats

Unsaturated fats increase the level of HDLs and decrease the level of LDLs in your blood, meaning eating more of them should result in less plaque accumulating in your blood vessels.

There are two types of unsaturated fat: monounsaturated and polyunsaturated. Oils, nuts, seeds, and oily fish contain each type in varying amounts. There are more specific examples on page 42.

A diet higher in unsaturated fat reduces the risk of cardiovascular disease. Current research also indicates that increasing your consumption of polyunsaturated fats, while decreasing your intake of carbohydrates and saturated fat (next page) can improve insulin sensitivity.

Saturated fats

Eating too much saturated fat can prevent your liver from removing LDLs from your blood, therefore causing the accumulation of harmful plaque. For this reason, saturated fats are associated with a greater risk of cardiovascular disease.

However, saturated fats are not all bad, they can be beneficial if consumed in moderation. They are a source of energy, are involved in hormone production, and contain vitamins A, D, E, and K2.

They are typically solid at room temperature and are found in dairy products, certain oils, and fatty meats. In dairy products, the more saturated fat the product has, generally the thicker it is.

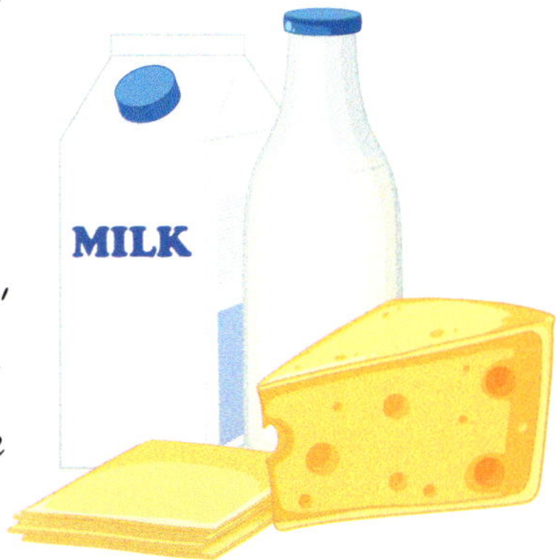

Trans fats

Trans fats can cause an increase in the LDL levels in the blood AND prevent the liver from removing LDLs from the blood, making them more harmful than saturated fats.

Trans fats are often found in vegetable oils repeatedly heated to a high temperature, fast foods, pastries, biscuits, and cakes. These are known as industrially produced trans fats and are the most harmful! These are the fats I recommend being particularly mindful of, as they seem to only have a negative effect.

In small amounts, trans fats can also be found in the fat of meat and dairy products. However, those listed in the paragraph above are far more harmful for your health.

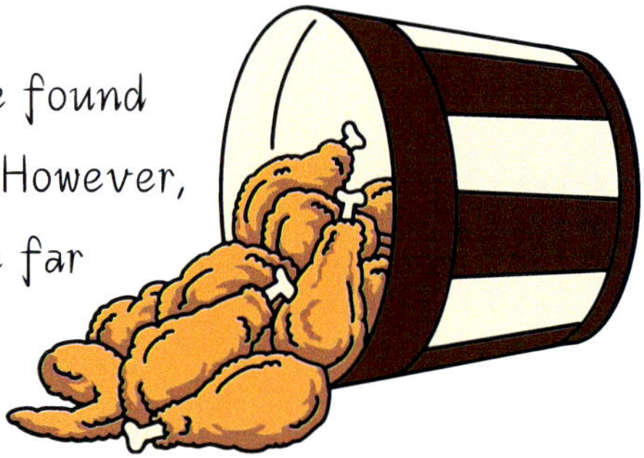

Fat examples

This table highlights different foods and the types of fat that they predominantly contain.

Monounsaturated	Polyunsaturated	Saturated	Trans
• Olive oil	• Flax seed oil	• Milk	• Vegetable oils heated to high temperatures repeatedly (e.g. deep fat fryers)
• Olives	• Flax seeds	• Yoghurt	• Pastries
• Sesame oil	• Sunflower oil	• Cheese	• Biscuits
• Rapeseed oil	• Sunflower seeds	• Butter	• Cakes
• Peanut oil	• Corn oil	• Cream	• Meat and dairy products (in small amounts)
• Peanuts	• Soybean oil	• Ice cream	
• Peanut butter	• Soybeans and edamame	• Fatty meats	
• Avocado	• Oily fish (e.g. salmon & mackerel)	• Processed meats	
• Almonds	• Walnuts	• Lard	
• Almond butter	• Chia seeds	• Palm oil	
• Pecans		• Palm kernel oil	
• Cashews		• Coconut oil	
• Hazelnuts		• Ghee	
• Pistachios			

When you are heating oil and it begins to smoke, this is a sign that the oil is losing its nutritional value, and is becoming toxic. Therefore, my recommendation is to cook at lower temperatures when possible.

Certain oils, like rapeseed oil, can reach higher temperatures before they begin to smoke, in comparison to olive oil. Therefore, you could make a stir fry with rapeseed oil and use raw olive oil on a salad, for example.

Top tip: air-fryers can allow you to cook at lower temperatures with less oil!

It is also important to avoid reheating the same cooking oil as this can further increase it's toxicity. This is in large part why fast food can be so harmful, because oil is often reused in deep fat friers.

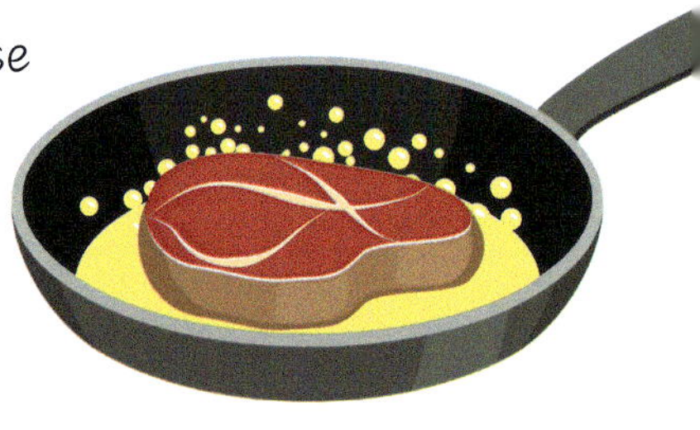

Protein

Protein consumption is important for repairing muscle and tissue, and regulating hormones, enzymes, and antibodies. Adding protein to meals can also reduce blood sugar spikes.

Proteins are made of amino acids, which are like little building blocks - the composition of which will dictate what the protein is for.

It is important to eat protein often, and with enough variety to include all of the amino acids that the body requires. There are nine 'essential amino acids' that cannot be made by the body.

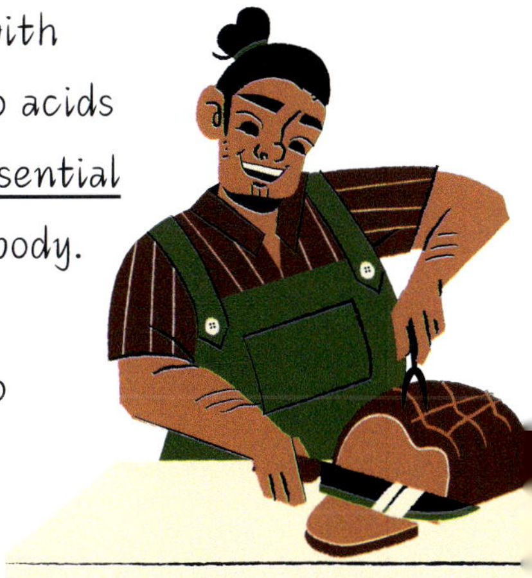

Proteins that contain all 9 essential amino acids are known as complete proteins, and those that don't are incomplete proteins.

Protein

Complete proteins give us all of the essential amino acids that the body requires, though it is still good to eat a variety of proteins, both complete and incomplete. If you are vegan or vegetarian, it is especially important to eat a variety of proteins.

Incomplete protein	Complete protein
All beans, peas, and lentils	Fish, poultry, pork, lamb, and beef
Most wholegrains and vegetables	Soy products, quinoa, chia seeds, and buckwheat
All nuts and most seeds	Eggs and dairy products

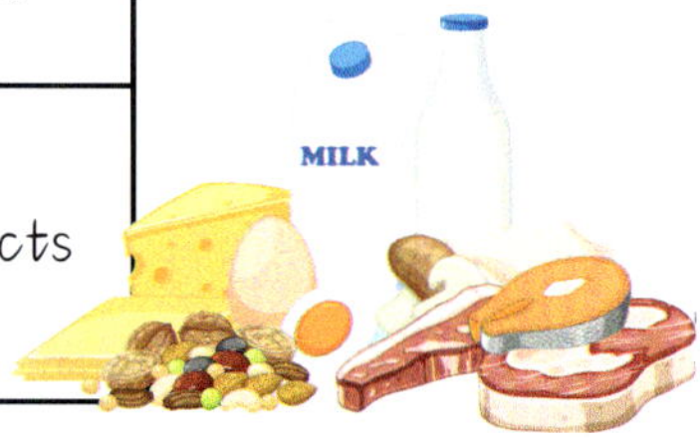

Antioxidants

Antioxidants are very powerful compounds which can improve various aspects of your health. They are shown to be capable of improving your body's response to insulin, which can help reduce your risk of developing type 2 diabetes.

They can also lower your risk of developing cardiovascular disease, inflammation (page 140), oxidative stress (page 143), and high blood pressure, as well as improve gut health (page 145), and skin health.

Antioxidant rich food and drinks include: walnuts, pecans, chestnuts, dark chocolate, berries, pomegranate, spinach, rosemary, bay leaves, cinnamon, cumin, and herbal teas like ginger, peppermint, chamomile, and hibiscus.

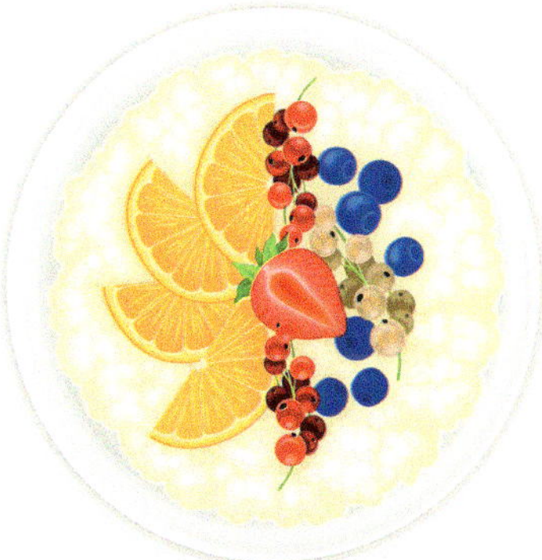

Snacking

The table below provides suggestions for changes you could make to your snacking habits. However, there is no such thing as a perfect snack, just better ones. It is important to pay attention to the snack choice, frequency, and portion size.

Snacks	Alternative suggestions
Fried potato crisps	Baked, wholegrain, vegetable, hummus, or lentil crisps, pea snacks, popcorn, nuts, and seeds
Biscuits and cakes	Home baked goods, oat cakes, rice cakes, lentil cakes or porridge with fruit and nuts
Milk or white chocolate	Dark chocolate
Sweets	Fresh/dried fruit, and yoghurt covered fruit or nuts
Ice cream	Yoghurt with toppings

Processed foods

When food is made, the further it strays from its original form, and the more additives that are added to the product - the more processed that food becomes. For example, cooked chicken is more processed than raw chicken. However, chicken nuggets, containing an assortment of additives, are even more processed because they have strayed further from the raw chicken.

Ultra processed foods have been shown to contribute to the development of type 2 diabetes, cardiovascular disease, certain forms of cancer, lung illnesses, inflammation, poor gut health, and obesity.

Remember, not all processed foods are bad, it is about finding those which will benefit you, rather than harm you, and this section can help.

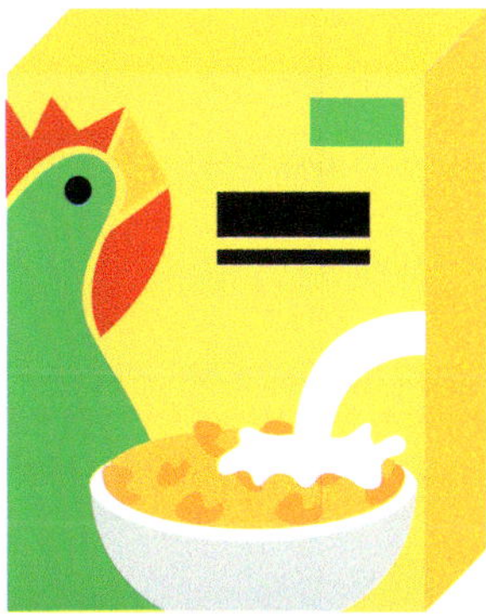

Reading food labels

Food labels are notoriously difficult to interpret. There are so many numbers, the font size is often too small, and the phrasing can be confusing. However, despite the difficulty, it is important to check the products you are buying so that you can avoid those which may cause you harm.

In most cases, food that you make from scratch will be better for your health. However, reading food labels can help you make healthy swaps for the ingredients and foods you buy regularly.

My advice would be to start by making minor adjustments to the staples of your diet, which you eat on a daily basis. These foods will have the greatest impact on your health because you eat them most frequently.

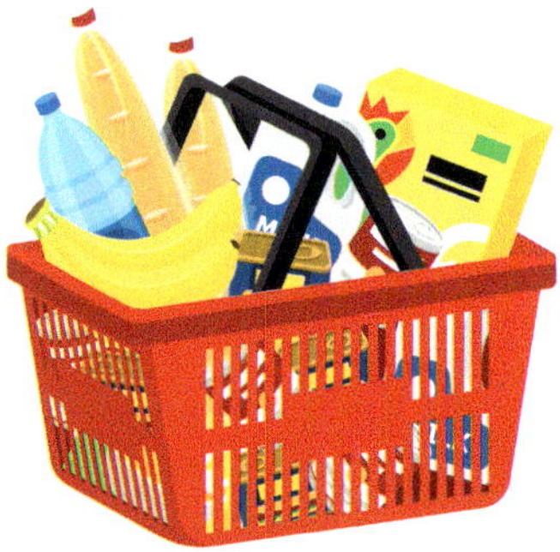

Natural sweeteners

Natural sweeteners like Maltitol, Xylitol, and Erythritol are known as Polyols. They are derived from fruits and plants and commonly used in baked goods and chocolate bars.

Foods which contain these sweeteners might make an effective swap for <u>some</u> people. In comparison to sugar; they are better for your teeth, lower in calories, and have a low GI. They also have pre-biotic properties and can improve gut health (page 145).

However, polyols can exacerbate gastrointestinal issues like IBS, and often have a laxative effect. Therefore, when introducing them to your diet, look out for any unpleasant symptoms.

Stevia

Stevia seems to be the golden child of natural sweeteners at the moment. According to some of the current research; pure stevia can reduce inflammation and blood pressure; it is better for your teeth than sugar, contains no calories, and has no effect on blood sugar.

Some individuals report that stevia can cause bloating and nausea, but research does not indicate that this is common.

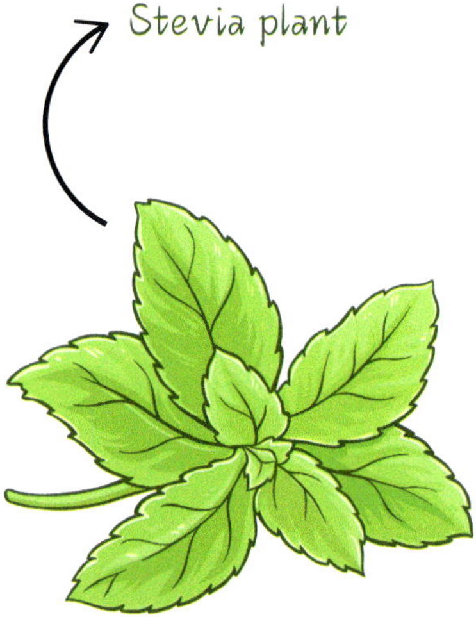

However, there is a difference between pure stevia, and a stevia blend, which may contain polyols (mentioned on page 54), and can cause gastrointestinal issues. Therefore, you should look at the ingredients.

The nutrition label

This is a typical nutrition label for a supermarket own-brand cheddar cheese, in the UK.

1	2	3	4	5
Typical values	100g	Per 30g serving	% based on RI for average adult	RI for average adult
Energy	1725kJ 416 kcal	517kJ 125kcal	6%	8400kJ 2000 kcal
Total fat	34.9g	10.5g	15%	70g
Saturated fat	21.7g	6.5g	33%	20g
Carbohydrates	0g	0g	0%	260g
of which sugars	0g	0g	0%	90g
Fibre	0g	0g	0%	30g
Protein	25.4g	7.6g	15%	50g
Salt	1.8g	0.54g	9%	6g

Traffic light system

These numbers dictate the colours for the traffic light system. The colours indicate whether a product contains high, medium or low amounts of fat, saturated fat, sugar, and salt, per 100g or 100ml. Use column 2 on page 56 to compare values.

	Low	Medium	High
Total fats	0 - 3g	3g - 17.5g	17.5g +
Saturates	0 - 1.5g	1.5g - 5g	5g +
Sugar	0 - 5g	5g - 22.5g	22.5g +
Salt	0 - 0.3g	0.3g - 1.5g	1.5g +

Per 100g or 100ml

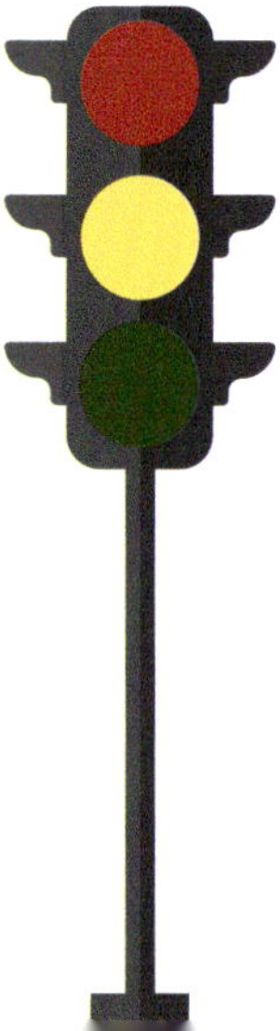

Traffic light system

There are a few things to be aware of when it comes to the traffic light system;

1. It is not used on all food packagings, so you might need to check for yourself.
2. The amber column is very broad.
3. It doesn't indicate how high into the red something can go.
4. If it is high in total fat but low in saturated fat, it mainly contains the healthier unsaturated fat - so red may not be bad.

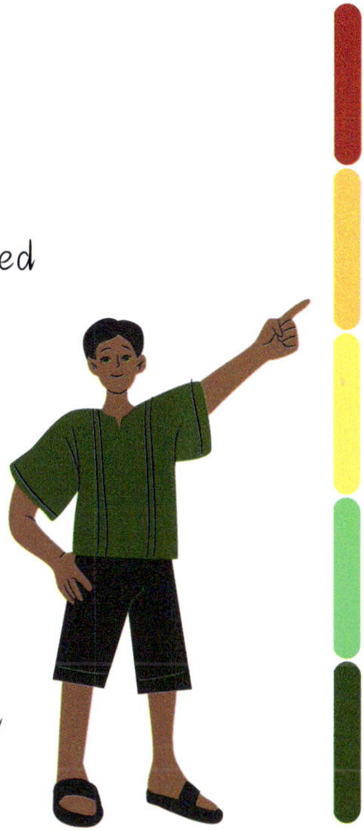

The traffic light system is useful for comparing food products and understanding whether they are proportionally better or worse for you. However, it is important to understand the nuances.

The traffic light system is useful. However, if you are having a portion, you are likely having more or less than 100g. The cheddar cheese example, on page 56, has a portion size of 30g.

Therefore, we use columns 3, 4, and 5 to understand the portion size. Column 3 shows you how much of each nutrient, and how much energy is in the portion. Column 4 shows how much this portion will contribute to an average adult's daily intake of food, which can be seen in column 5.

For example, this portion contains 6.5g of saturated fat - which is 33% of an average adult's daily intake of saturated fat - of 20g. This can help you understand how much is really in a portion. This example is highlighted in blue.

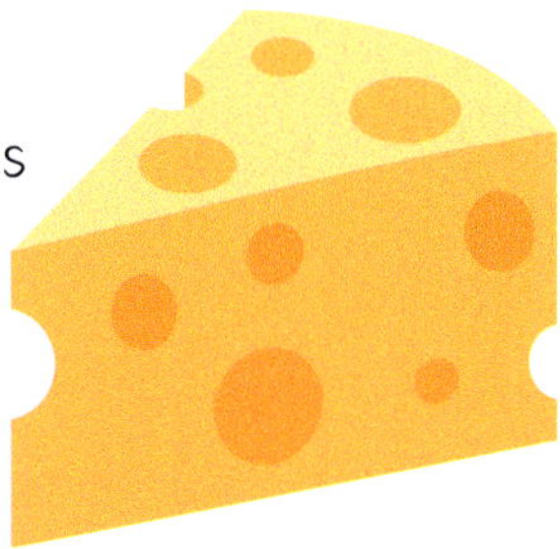

Front nutrition label

Alternatively, on the front of the packaging for certain foods, there will be a series of boxes like the ones below. These give you the same information as columns 3 and 4 on page 56.

The numbers on top indicate how many calories, and grams of fat, saturated fat, sugar, and salt are present in that portion of food. Sometimes the boxes will be coloured green, amber, or red. Other times they won't, like in the example below.

The percentage tells us how much this portion will contribute to an average adult's daily intake of food.

This portion contains 12% of an average adults daily salt intake!

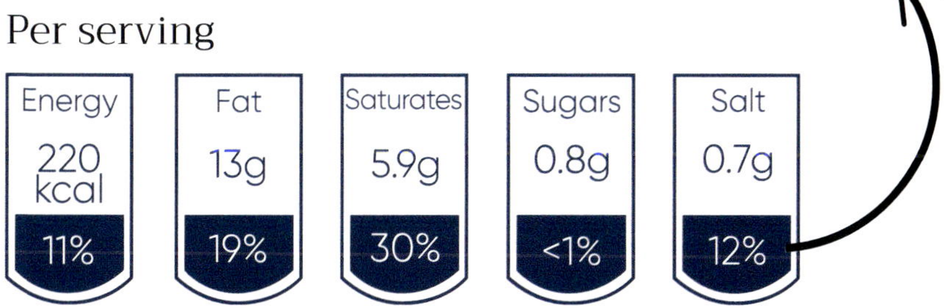
Per serving
Energy
220 kcal
11%
Fat
13g
19%
Saturates
5.9g
30%
Sugars
0.8g
<1%
Salt
0.7g
12%

Salt intake

Excessive salt consumption contributes to high blood pressure, and the risk of cardiovascular disease, heart attacks, and strokes. This is because the sodium in salt increases the amount of water in your blood. This means there will be more liquid in your bloodstream, which will push against the inner walls of your blood vessels with more force - or <u>pressure</u>.

It is important to check the products that you are buying for their salt content. It is commonly used as a preservative and many products will have more salt than you'd expect; like sauces and seasonings. Additionally, salt that you add to food both before and after cooking makes a big difference.

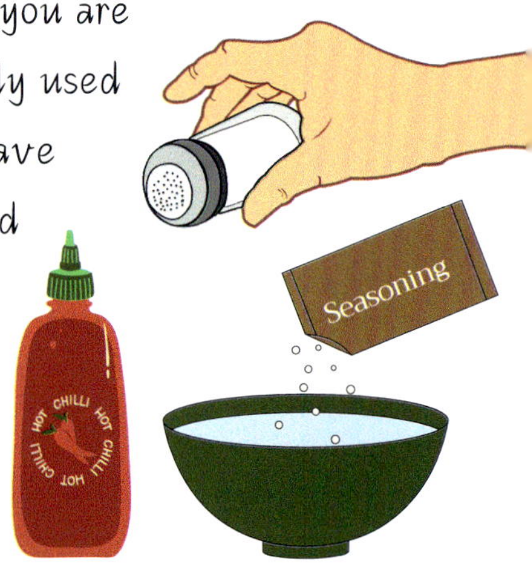

Hydration

When blood sugar is elevated, the body gets rid of excess sugar through urine. Hence why diabetics constantly feel thirsty and urinate frequently.

Therefore, chronic dehydration can contribute to the development of type 2 diabetes, because the body isn't able to expel glucose from the body as effectively. Drinking more water can improve the way your body processes sugar in the blood.

Furthermore, water is essential for all forms of life. Water allows biochemical reactions to take place inside of your body cells and is important for transportation of nutrients, temperature regulation, and lubrication of joints. I can't stress enough how important water is.

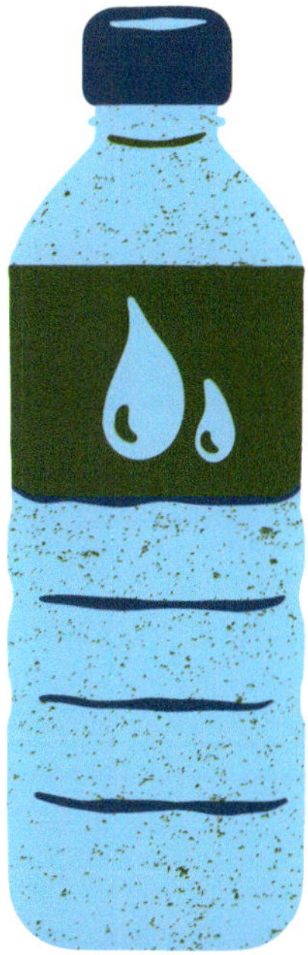

Hydration

Water alone is hydrating. However, tea, coffee, squash, flavoured water, soup, and infused water are also hydrating, and all contribute to your total water consumption.

It is recommended that people consume 1.5 to 2 litres of water per day in total. I'd recommend continuously drinking throughout the day, taking small sips whenever you are able. If you forget to drink water or you don't often feel thirsty, I'd also suggest setting an hourly alarm.

I should point out that drinks like squash and flavoured water may have additional sugar or sweeteners. Infusing water with fruit or something like cucumber might make a better long-term solution.

Portions

In my experience, portion size and composition are often overlooked, however, this is very likely to affect your health, because you eat portions of food <u>every</u> day.

When considering your portions, you could try arranging your plate like the pie chart to the right. This is an efficient way of controlling your intake of carbohydrates, while consuming an adequate amount of protein and fibre.

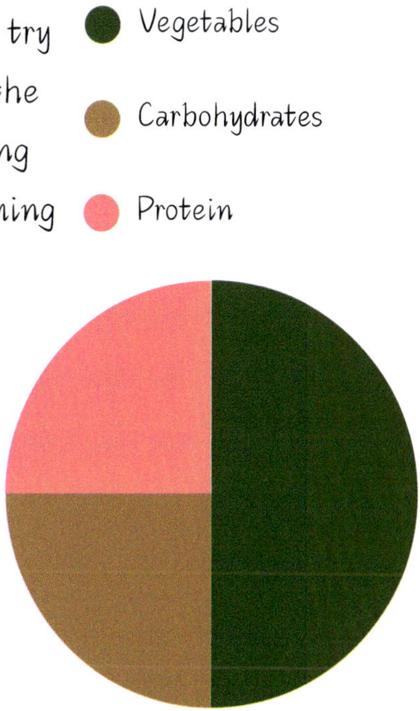

This is not the "perfect portion", it is simply a <u>guideline</u>, and an effective way of becoming more aware of your portions. You could follow this guideline as often as you like, and there are even plates you can buy which match the pie chart.

Food choices

The benefit of the guideline on the previous page is that you can adjust it to suit you and your preferences.

You could also start adding foods which offer multiple benefits for your health. For example, oats, nuts, seeds, and beans all contain protein and fibre. As a result, they are lower glycemic index foods, which are beneficial for managing blood sugar and appetite. Therefore, you get four benefits from adding just one of those foods to your diet.

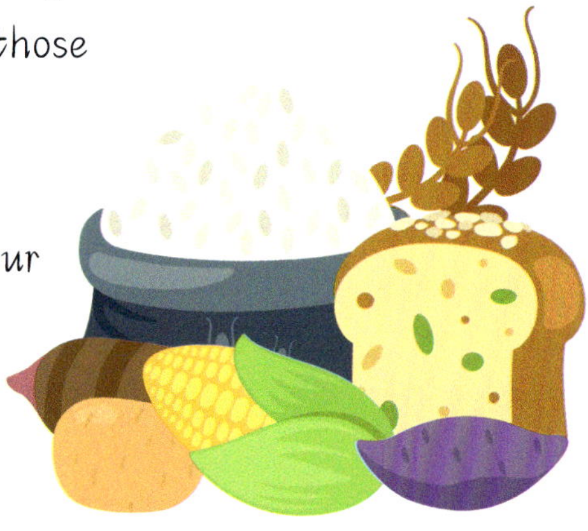

Adding these multi-benefit foods to your diet can help you improve your health with small and simple changes.

Portion size

When considering the size of your portion, you can use your hands as a guide. As shown on the bottom right - if you hold your hands side by side with your palms flat and fingers together - that is theoretically the size of your portion on a plate. If you then curve your hands, that is a bowl.

This may not be a perfect system, but it does give you a baseline to make changes. If you attempt this and find yourself overly hungry and snacking, you can make your portions slightly bigger until you find your goldilocks amount.

Portion size can help you control your blood sugar, and your bodyweight, especially if you do this in tandem with other changes.

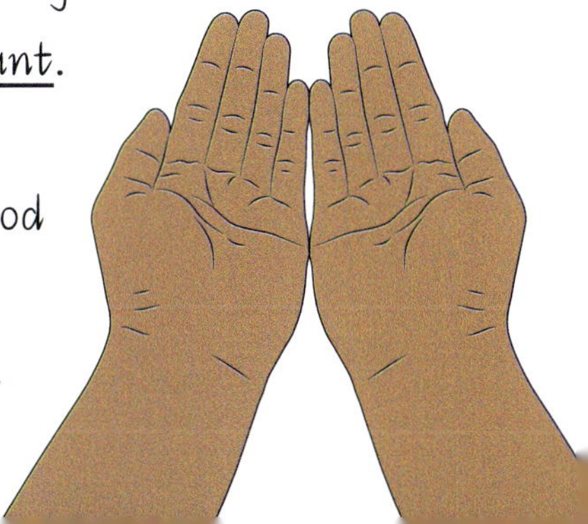

Calories

Calories (or kcal) are neither good nor bad, they simply represent how much energy exists inside of food. High calorie foods can be beneficial, just as low calorie foods can cause issues, but it is your consumption of food overall which will dictate whether you gain or lose weight.

Carbohydrates and proteins both contain 4 calories per gram. Fats on the other hand, contain 9 calories per gram. Hence why foods like nuts and avocado, which contain high amounts of unsaturated fat, are high in calories.

Fortunately, you don't need to count calories to manage your weight. I recommend trialling new portion sizes and making food swaps so that you can better manage your energy balance.

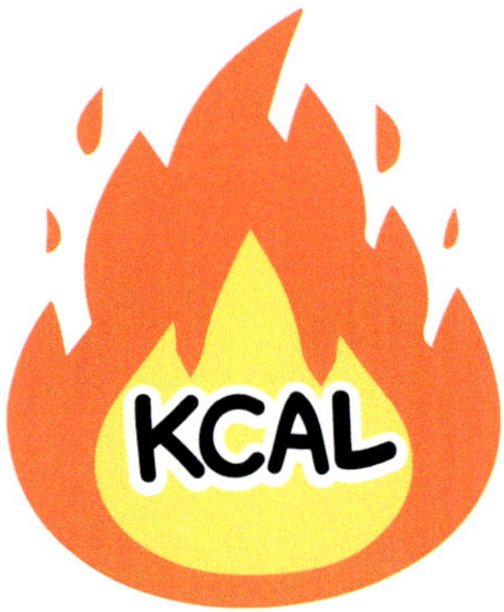

Energy balance

Energy balance refers to the amount of energy you are consuming and burning day-to-day. This is the mechanism which influences weight gain and weight loss.

Energy you consume will be in the form of food and drink and is usually measured in calories. The energy you burn is determined by your activity levels, and your Basal Metabolic Rate, or BMR.

Your BMR is the minimum number of calories your body requires to perform life-sustaining functions like breathing, blood circulation, and maintaining your body temperature. Essentially, it is the number of calories you require to survive if you did nothing at all.

BMR is dictated by:

- Genetics
- Gender
- Age
- Body composition
- General health

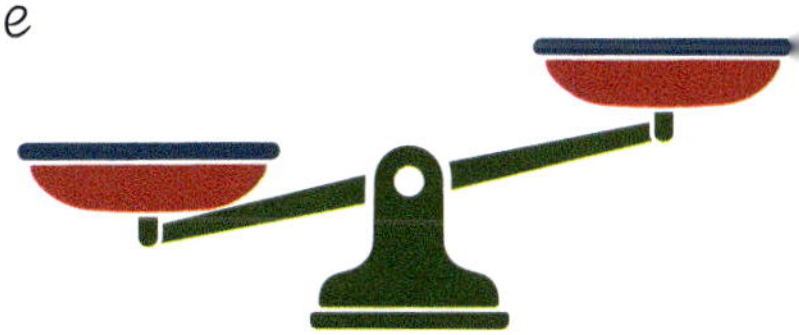

Weight change

On paper, it is simple. If you want to lose weight, you must consume fewer calories than you burn on a daily basis, so that you are in a calorie deficit. This can be achieved by controlling your portion sizes, eating less frequently, and exercising more.

However, not everybody reading this book must lose weight. If you want to gain weight, you must consume more calories than you burn on a daily basis, so that you are in a calorie surplus. This can be achieved by controlling your portion sizes, eating more frequently, and eating calorie dense food.

In reality, many people really struggle to lose weight.

If you would like to maintain your weight, you must eat an equal number of calories in comparison to the number that you burn.

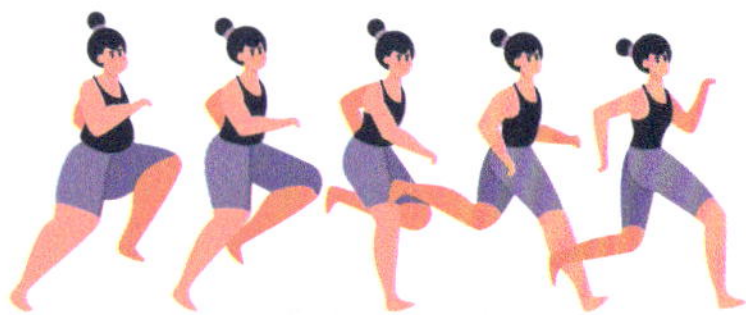

Weight change

Having excess body-fat makes your body more resistant to insulin, and therefore less capable of processing sugar in the blood. It is therefore important to make changes if you are carrying too much body fat - but it is also crucial to do so in a healthy way.

When stepping on the scale, it can be easy to beat yourself up for the number you see or don't see. Therefore, it is important to be objective.

If you can be objective about the results, whether positive or negative, then you can see what is working and what isn't. This can then help you take the next steps - like adjusting the food on your plate, or the size of your portion. If you just beat yourself up, it can be difficult to move forward positively.

Eating habits

Many people have had the same eating habits for a long time. Those eating habits affect your food choices, meal patterns, snack preferences, and portion sizes.

Changing those eating habits takes time and patience. However, I hope that this section has highlighted changes you can see yourself making.

Page 107 is about altering habits.

Keeping track of your eating habits can make you more aware of them, and give you a better understanding of why you eat the way that you do. Making a food diary, for example, is an effective way of analysing those habits so that you can make changes. Just don't expect them to happen overnight!

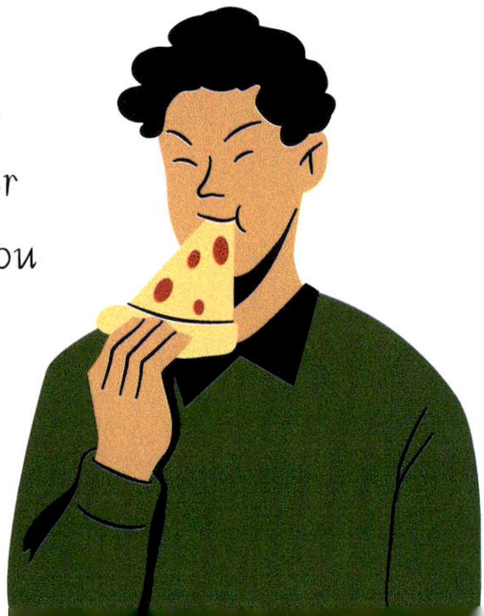

Food diary template

You can create a food diary using the template below. This can be used to track your current eating habits and any changes you are making.

	Breakfast	Lunch	Dinner	Snacks	Drinks	Changes
Monday						
Tuesday						
Wednesday						
Thursday						
Friday						
Saturday						
Sunday						

Reflection point 2

This is a list of suggestions based on the information from this section:

- Swap higher GI foods for lower GI foods.
- Make adjustments to the GI of your meals and snacks using the suggestions provided.
- Add a variety of fibre, healthy fats, proteins, and antioxidant rich foods to your diet.
- Cook at lower temperatures so that the oil doesn't smoke.
- Read food labels and look out for additives and high quantities of saturated fat, salt, and sugar.
- Drink 1.5-2 litres of water per day.
- Trial the recommended portion guideline.
- Work towards a healthy bodyweight.
- Try maintaining a food diary.

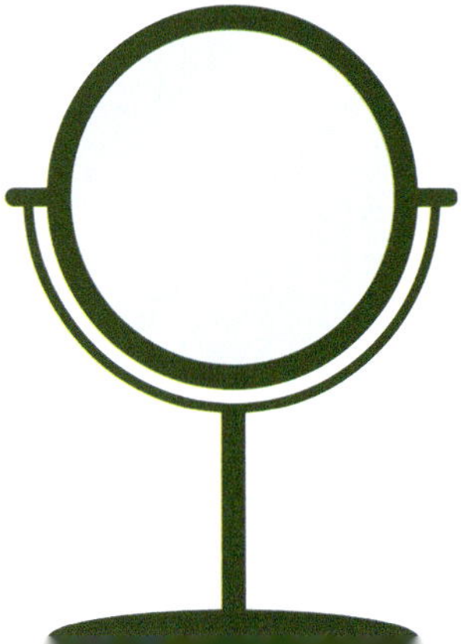

Section 3
EXERCISE AND PHYSICAL ACTIVITY

"We are what we repeatedly do. Excellence, then is not an act, but a habit."

— Aristotle

The history of exercise

Hippocrates (460-370 BC) and Galen (129-210 AD), mentioned on page 4, were two of the first to educate people on the importance of physical activity.

Hippocrates was the first physician in recorded history to prescribe exercise for a patient struggling with consumption (now known as Tuberculosis).

Galen was a physician for the gladiators and often recommended rehabilitation therapy and exercise regimes that he created himself. He also introduced the term 'polisarkia' - meaning too much food, and too little exercise when referring to obesity. Much of his work is still relevant and influential today.

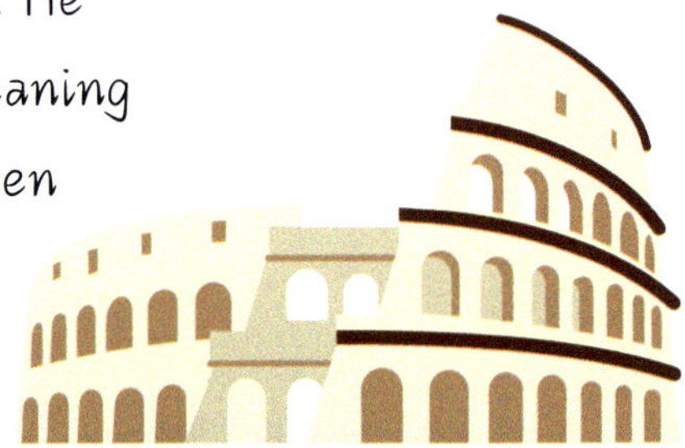

Physical activity

Physical activity has a dramatic effect on your health. It can reduce the risk of cardiovascular disease, cancers, and mental health disorders like anxiety and depression, as well as improve sleep and bone density.

On top of the benefits outlined above, exercise can also help you decrease your risk of developing type 2 diabetes.

Physical activity is classed as 'any bodily movement produced by skeletal muscles that requires energy expenditure'. Meaning, when we voluntarily use our muscles and move around, this counts as physical activity. You don't have to do "conventional" exercise to become more active.

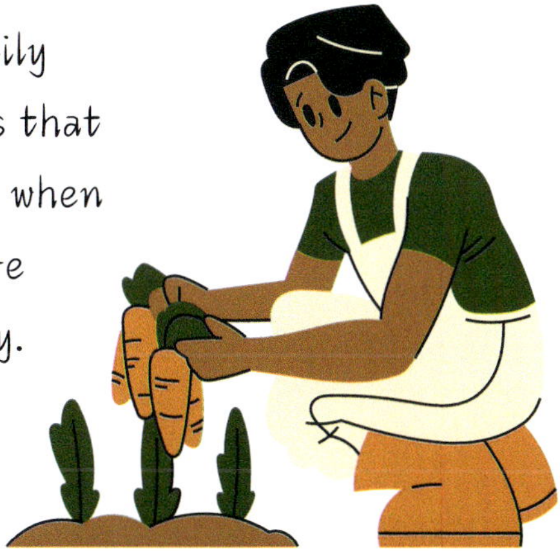

Activity and blood sugar

Exercise can influence your blood sugar immediately. When you exercise at a low intensity, like going for a moderate walk or doing chair exercises - your blood sugar should decrease.

However, when you exercise at high intensities - like doing an intense spin class - your blood sugar is likely to increase, to support the needs of the body. That doesn't mean you should avoid high intensity exercise, a good balance is key.

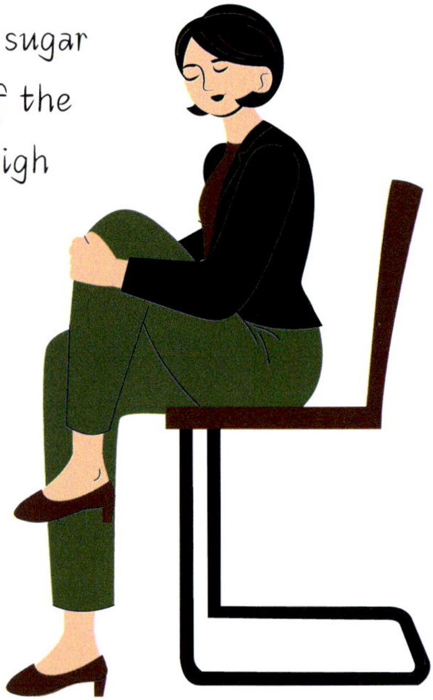

Additionally, by exercising more frequently, for longer durations, the body cells become more insulin sensitive. Therefore, even a small amount of exercise everyday, like a short walk, can help you control your blood sugar better in the long run.

Components of fitness

These are four important components of fitness;

- Cardiovascular fitness
- Muscular strength and endurance
- Flexibility
- Balance

Combined, these components affect every aspect of your health, and the way your body functions day-to-day. It is important to consider your gaps - the areas of your own fitness where you are lacking. If you don't use it, you will lose it.

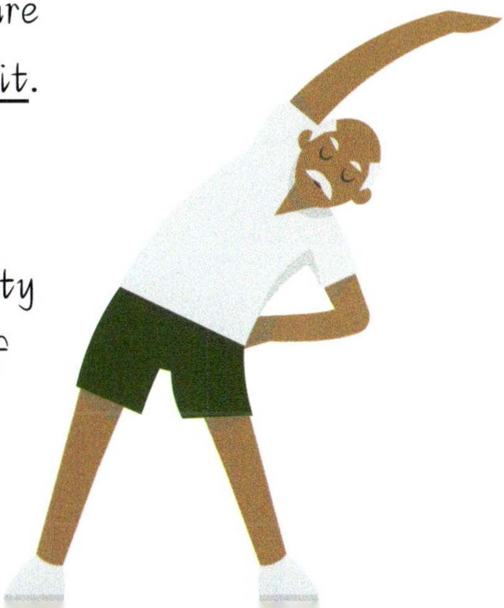

If you are lacking in one or more of these areas, that element of your physical ability will not improve and is likely to decline if you do not intervene and make a change. Fortunately, small changes go a long way.

Cardiovascular fitness

Cardiovascular fitness is a measure of how well the heart, lungs, and circulatory system get blood to your muscles, to give them oxygen.

Cardiovascular exercises are those which cause your heart rate and breathing rate to rise, and more blood to circulate around the body. At low or high intensities, these exercises can improve the strength of your heart, the efficiency of your lungs, and cleanliness of your blood vessels.

Daily actitivties like washing up or walking the dog contribute to your activity levels!

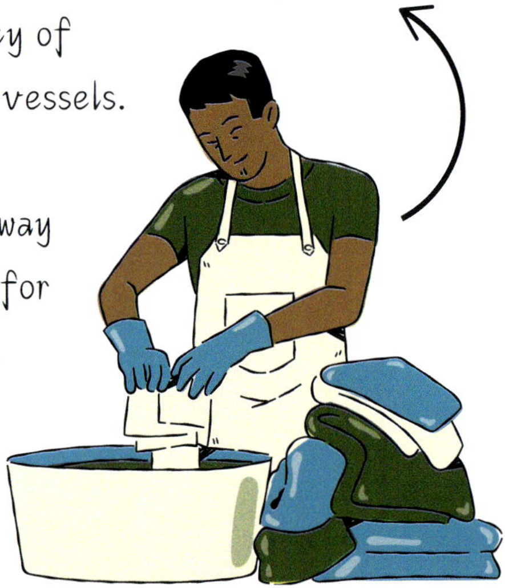

Taking part in sport can be an enjoyable way of making improvements, as well as going for walks, martial arts, gardening, housework, exercise videos, or finding local exercise groups and clubs.

Muscular strength and endurance

Muscular strength and endurance refers to the amount of force you can generate with your muscles, and the length of time they can perform an action. If you have found that your ability to move yourself and everyday objects has declined, I would suggest doing resistance exercises to counter this issue and improve on it.

Resistance exercises involve repetitive movements which force you to contract your muscles against an external force.

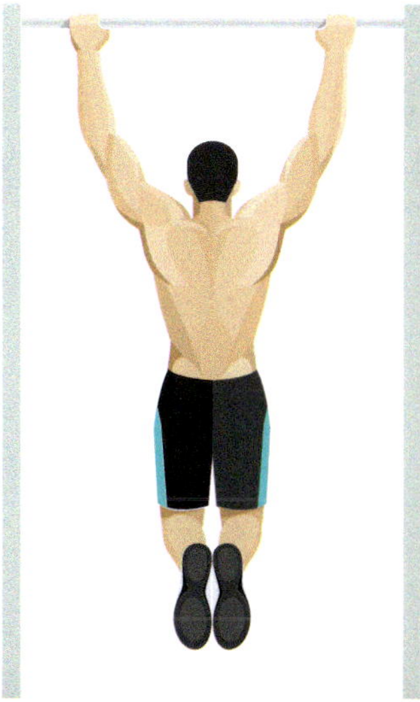

You could do body weight exercises like push-ups and lunges, or use free weights, machines, and resistance bands. Alternatively, sports like rugby and swimming are very effective and can improve cardiovascular fitness as well.

Flexibility

Flexibility refers to your ability to move parts of your body through the full range of motion at a joint. For example, your ability to rotate your arm around your shoulder in a full circle, or completely straighten and bend your knee.

The structure of a joint will determine its range of motion, as will your ability to stretch muscles and tendons (soft tissue which connects muscle to bone), and the health of your ligaments (hard tissue which connects bone to bone).

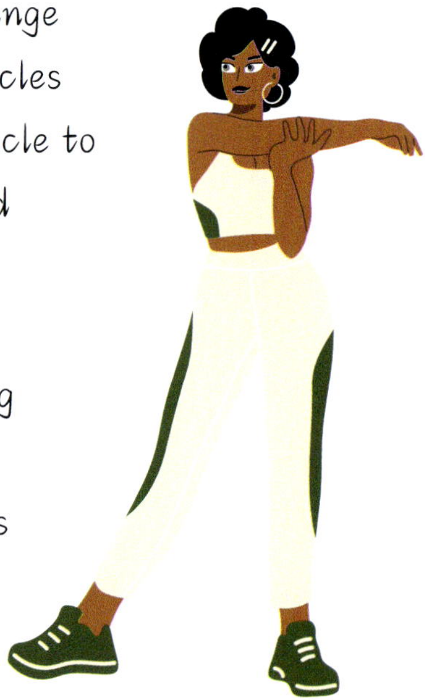

Do you often feel stiff and achy? Stretching for just a short duration daily or weekly can improve your mobility and relieve you of this issue, as well as decrease your risk of injury. I'd recommend yoga or chair-based routines.

Balance

Balance refers to the stability of your body, and your ability to maintain your centre of gravity.

Balance is a key example of the 'use it or lose it' principle. How many people have you encountered in your life, who rely on support to move around without falling? Unfortunately, this will be the case for many people unless they actively attempt to improve their balance.

Balance is a key indicator of longevity!

By practicing movements which challenge you to maintain your upright position, you can improve your balance. You could practice standing on 1 leg for 30 seconds a day. Alternatively, yoga and pilates can help improve balance, as well as flexibility.

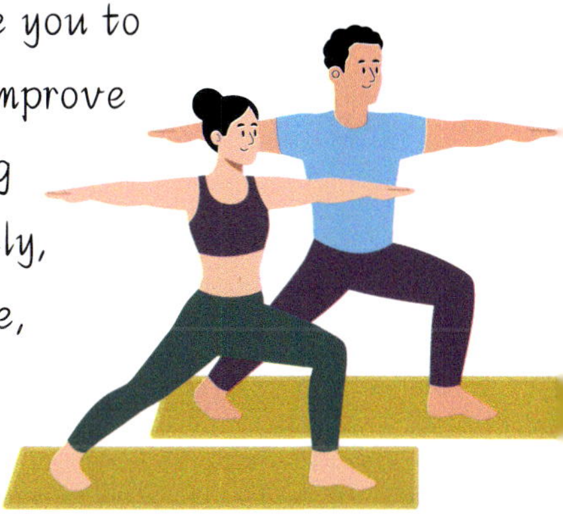

Activity and weight

On page 68, I explain energy balance, which tells us that our weight is dictated by the amount of energy we consume and burn over time.

Exercising can help you to lose weight because you can burn more calories than if you are sedentary - meaning it is easier to achieve a calorie deficit. However, for people who do not want to lose weight, it is still important to be active.

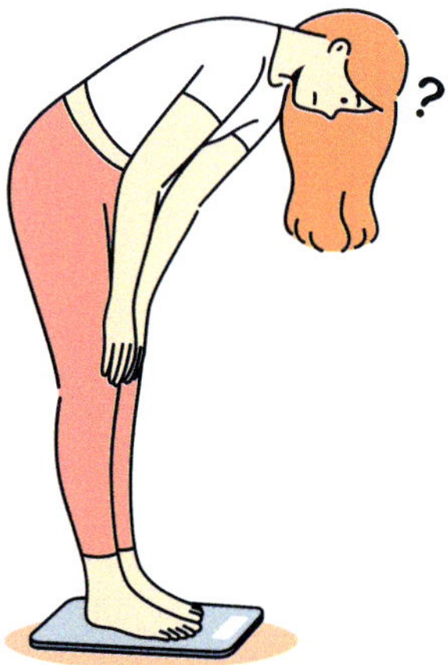

Exercise alone doesn't guarantee weight loss, it also depends on your food intake (page 68). Exercise can even cause your weight to increase if you are gaining muscle. Therefore, it is important to not solely rely on the numbers, but also consider how you feel and your shape.

Activity and mental health

Activity is directly related to your mental health.

When you exercise, dopamine (page 105), serotonin, and endorphins are released in the brain, which can improve your mood and mental state. These are just some of the positive changes that take place when you are physically active.

Exercise is consistently shown to reduce levels of stress, anxiety, and depression. It can also help people struggling with addiction, and improve memory.

Many people no longer live in a world where they need to be physically active to survive. That doesn't mean that exercise can't improve your health and happiness.

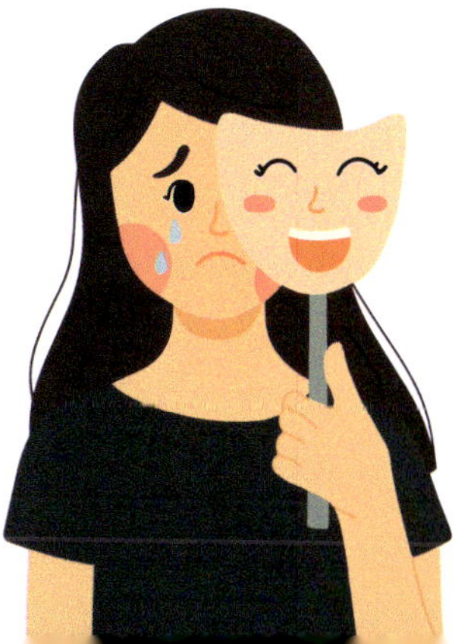

Recommendations

The NHS and World Health Organisation recommend that adults do at least 150 minutes of moderate exercise, and 75 minutes of vigorous exercise every week. Or a combination of both. Additionally, adults should do resistance exercises two times per week.

In reality, you should adjust your exercise levels according to your current ability. I'd recommend adding exercises and activities to your daily life so that you can form healthier habits and find enjoyable ways of exercising.

You could try standing on one leg while brushing your teeth, walking to work from a further bus stop everyday, or even taking the stairs instead of the lift or escalator.

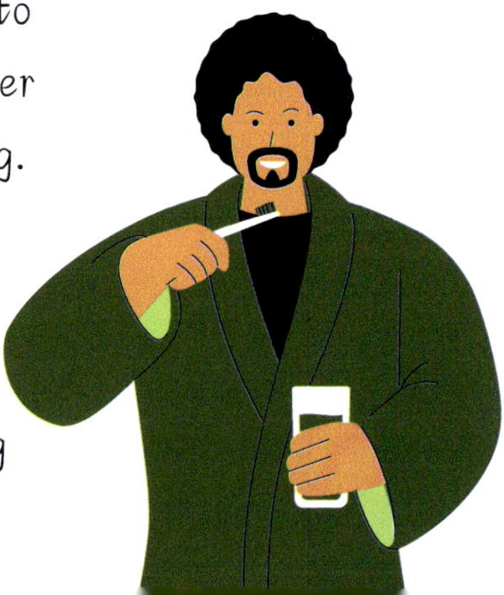

The FITT principle

If you want to become more physically active, I would suggest using the FITT principle to do so. This is a framework which can help you understand your activity levels and make adjustments.

FITT stands for:

- Frequency - how often you are active.
- Intensity - how intensely you are exercising.
- Type - the types of exercises you are doing.
- Time - how much time you are active for.

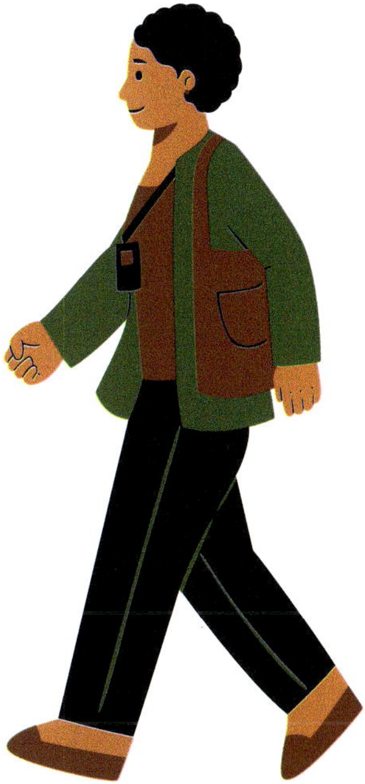

This is a very useful tool that is often used by fitness professionals to help people exercise more. On the next page is a series of questions which can help you understand each of these elements so you can take the next steps.

Applying FITT

Answer the questions below to assess your current level of activity, and understand where you can make improvements. <u>It isn't necessary to make extreme changes</u>. Just five more minutes a day, or one extra bout of exercise per week can make a difference!

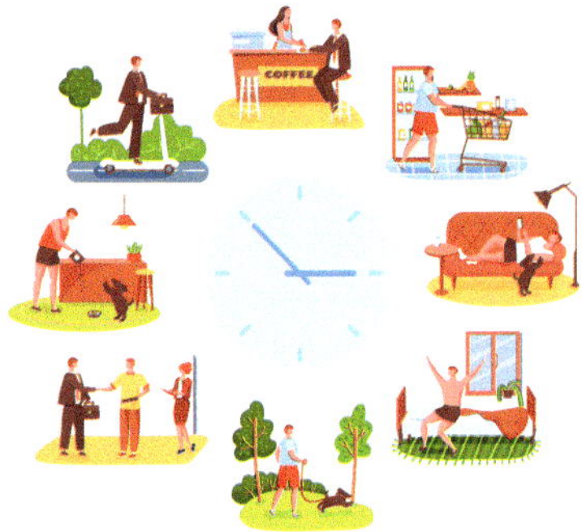

Frequency	How often am I active throughout the day/week? Am I be able to add to this?
Intensity	Do I exercise at lower and higher intensities? How can I vary the intensity?
Type	What types of exercises am I doing? Do I have any gaps in my physical ability?
Time	How much time am I active for during the day/week? Am I able to add to this?

Reflection point 3

This is a list of suggestions based on the information from this section:

- Do light physical activity or exercises, such as: taking a walk, doing chair exercises, or housework, to manage your blood sugar.
- Start varying the intensity of exercises you do, where you can, from moderate to intense.
- Look for gaps in your physical ability and include new exercises which address them.
- Exercise with the intention of controlling your bodyweight.
- Exercise with the intention of improving your mental state.
- Make small changes and recognise your limits.
- Use the FITT principle to help make changes.

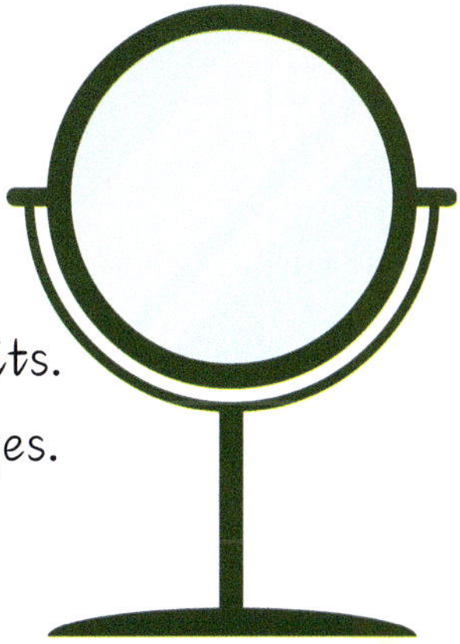

Section 4
STRESS, HABITS, AND THOUGHTS

"It's not stress that kills us, it is our reaction to it."

— Hans Selye

Stress

Human beings are prone to experiencing stress for long and short durations, and for any number of reasons. Yet, we rarely take time to reflect on how it is affecting our health.

I like to say that stress is indiscriminate - it doesn't care about your particular situation. That isn't to say that your circumstances are not important, they are. Only that stress will wreak havoc on your health, regardless of the situation that is causing it.

Therefore, this section is all about recognising different forms of stress, the effect it has on humans generally, the ways in which it affects you as an individual, and how to deal with it in a healthier way.

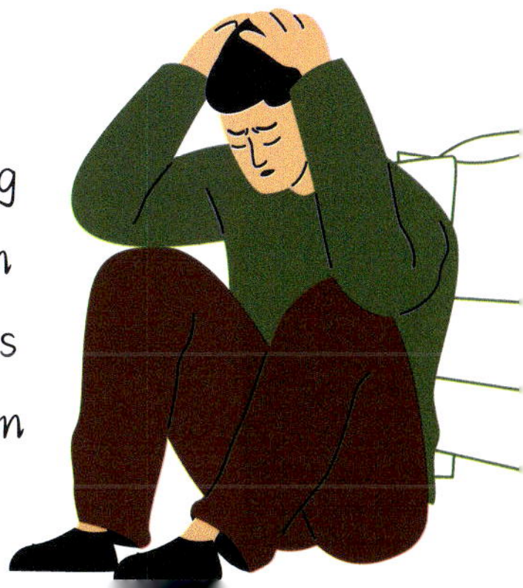

Stress research

During the 19th and early 20th centuries, the word 'stress' was used in engineering to describe how well a material could withstand external forces.

Between the 1930s and 1950s, a researcher named Hans Selye (1907 - 1982) began researching stress, but in relation to physiology. He studied the effect of different stressors on the physical states of rats. These stressors included cold exposure, exercise, injuries, and drugs.

Selye found that the rats would experience the same physiological changes, regardless of the type of stressor the rat was experiencing. This led him to define stress as "the non-specific response of the body to any demand placed upon it". Meaning, the stress response is general and universal.

Selye is known as the father of stress research.

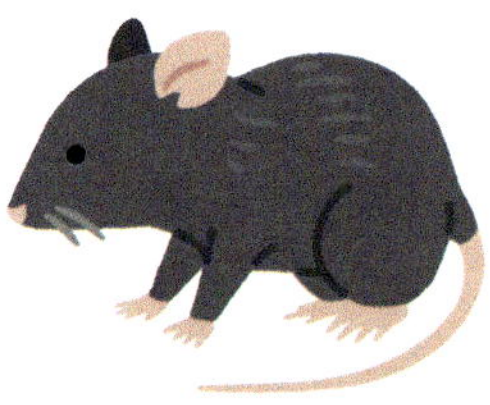

Fight or flight

The 'fight or flight' response was proposed by Professor Walter Cannon (1871 - 1945) in 1915. The theory suggests that humans experience general changes in their physical and mental states when they are in danger, or physically demanding situations, to ensure their survival.

This survival mechanism would have helped us to hunt, fight for territory, and escape predators.

There are more modern theories on stress, however, Hans Selye and Walter Cannon are pioneers in this area. They theorised and demonstrated that stress leads to changes and adaptations in the brain and body. Those changes and the effects they have on human health is what we will explore further in this section.

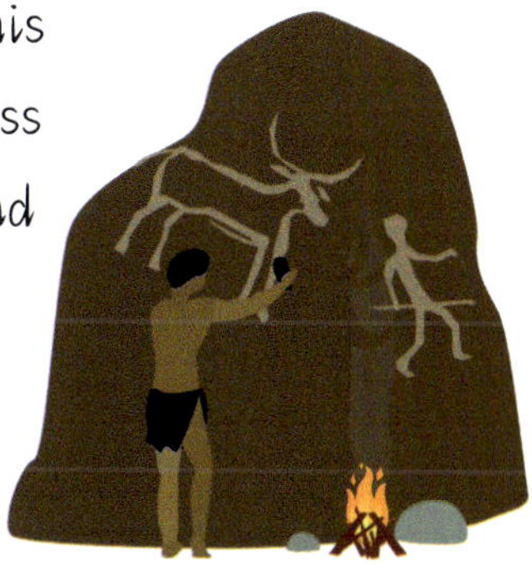

Acute stress

'Acute stress' refers to stress that we experience for short durations (minutes/hours). In this state, your hormones change; the levels of adrenaline, noradrenaline, and cortisol in your bloodstream increase, causing physiological and psychological changes, some of which are listed below. These changes occur in order to prepare you for action.

- Body temperature = increases
- Breathing rate = increases
- Blood pressure = increases
- Blood sugar = increases
- Heart rate = increases
- Digestion = decreases
- Alertness = increases
- Libido = decreases

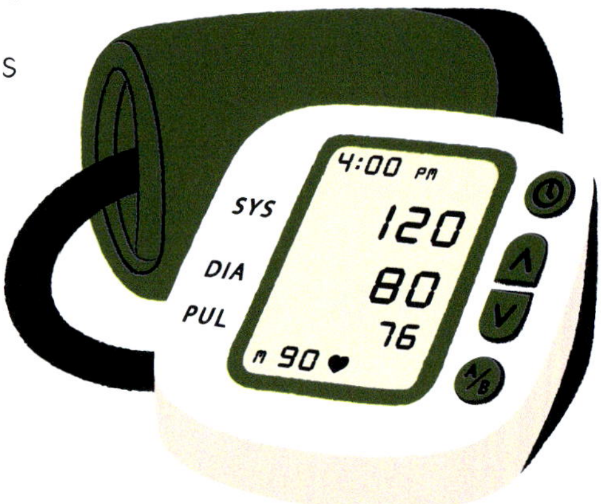

Chronic stress

Chronic stress develops when you experience on-going bouts of acute stress. If persistent, the physiological and psychological changes listed on the previous page can cause a number of health issues including: cardiovascular disease, inflammation, oxidative stress, a weakened immune system, poor gut health, and depression.

Additionally, acute stress causes your blood sugar to rise, meaning if you are chronically stressed, you have a higher chance of developing type 2 diabetes.

Chronic stress might be contributing to your health issues! For this reason, it is important to consider your stress levels and start paying attention to your stress symptoms.

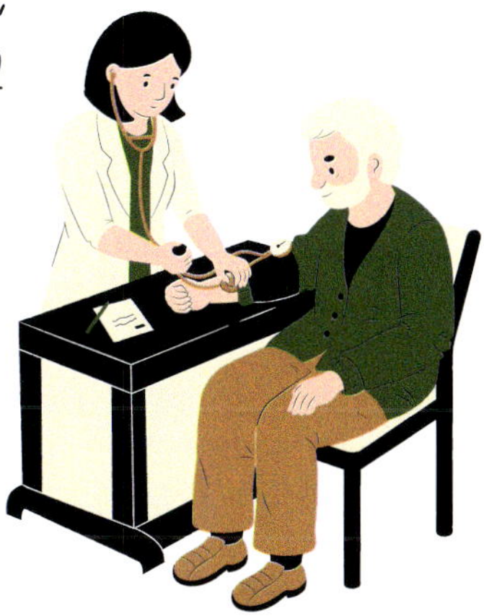

Stress symptoms

The changes listed on page 91 can explain your individual stress symptoms. For example, when a person is stressed and they sweat, it is because their body temperature increases.

Stress symptoms can include heart palpitations, a tight chest, nausea, fidgeting, shaking, sweating, feeling fixated, poor memory, hunger, difficulty sleeping, erectile dysfunction, irritability, pain, sadness, and anger. You may experience others.

These symptoms indicate that you are stressed, and if you don't do anything to address it, you may become chronically stressed. Therefore, it is important to recognise your symptoms so that you can reduce your stress levels before your health begins to decline.

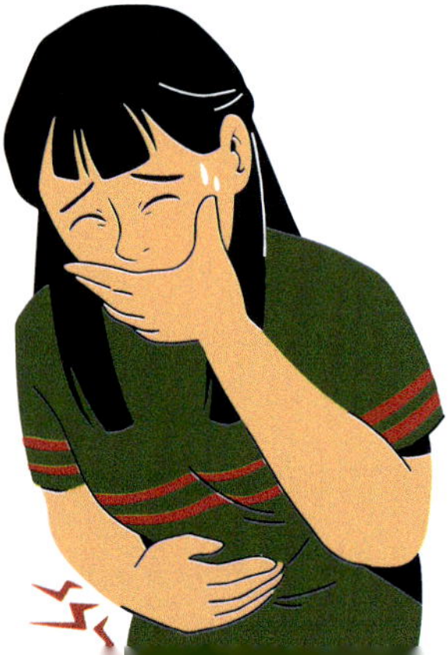

Internal stress

Often, the stress we experience is the result of our life situation and things happening around us. However, for many people, the stress they experience is the result of their own thoughts, worries, and perceptions.

Your mind and body are closely connected. For this reason, when you view something as a threat or problem, you are likely to experience acute stress, even if you are not in danger.

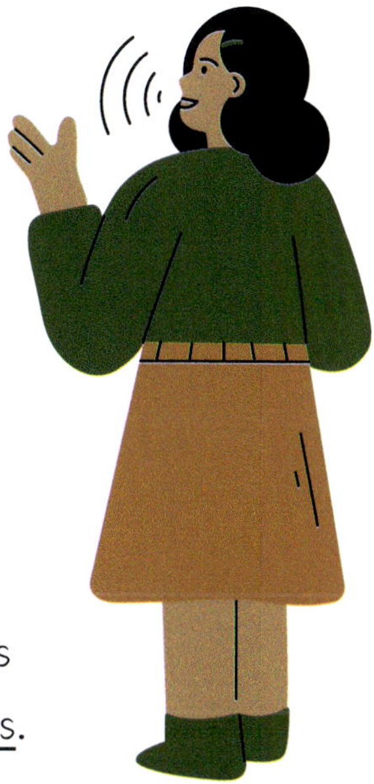

For example, if a person is afraid of public speaking - they might feel their heart rate and breathing rate rapidly increase. Whereas, another person who is accustomed to public speaking might feel no change. This demonstrates how our own perception can alter our stress levels.

Collectively, we spend a lot of time in our own heads, and that isn't always a pleasant place to be. It is worth considering how much time you spend up there, and whether you get caught in 'thought traps'. These are thoughts that keep you in your head, and prevent you from interacting with the world and reality.

This seems to be part of the human condition - we are built to analyse and strategise. However, if the way you think is negatively impacting your health, your stress levels, and perceptions of yourself, it might be worth making adjustments.

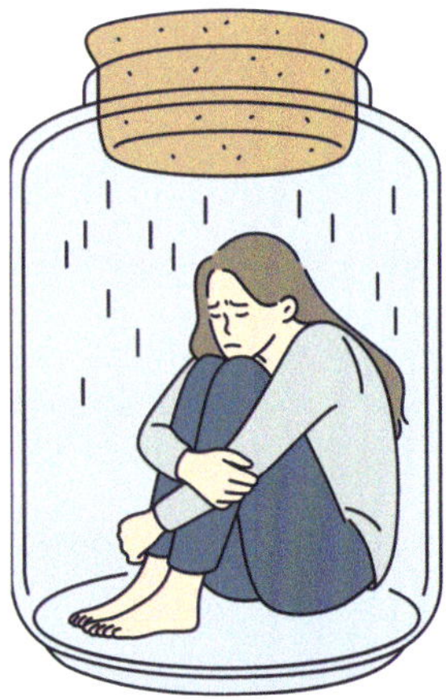

The next two pages contain common thought traps - acknowledging that you fall into these traps can help you break the cycle.

Rigid rules

- Setting yourself unrealistic rules, goals, and expectations, ultimately leading to stress and disappointment.

All or nothing

- Believing that things must be one way or another, and that there is no in-between.

Negative self-criticism

- Having thoughts about yourself that are unkind and counterproductive to your goals.

Labelling

- Labelling your entire character based on small and specific aspects of your personality.

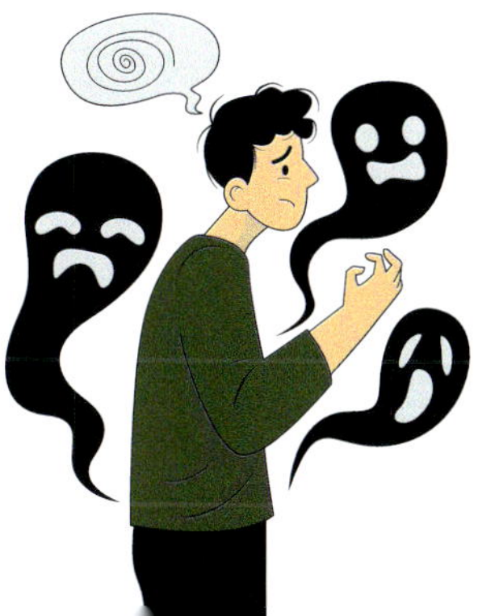

Catastrophising

- Expecting the worst possible outcomes.

Problem searching

- Looking for, or creating problems where they may not exist.

Excessive planning

- Planning every aspect of the future to escape the present. This can lead to disappointment and prevent you from moving forward.

Living in the past

- Consistently reliving past experiences and scenarios. This can also prevent you from moving forward.

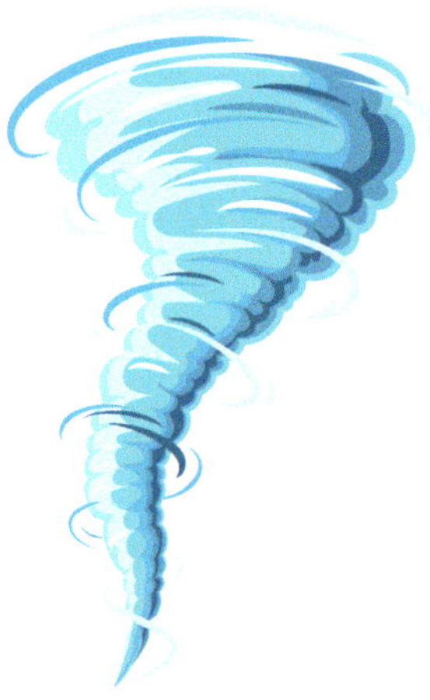

Getting out of your head

Getting out of your head and adjusting the way you think is a difficult task. It requires patience and compassion. Simply recognising the way that you think is a positive step.

You could try taking 'thought breaks'. This involves directing your attention to activities that help you break thought patterns, so that you can return to them with a fresh perspective. For example, you could read a book, speak with a friend, or go for a walk.

Communicating your thoughts to another person, or simply getting them out of your head, could help you break thought patterns as well. You could record yourself thinking out loud, or write your thoughts in a journal or diary.

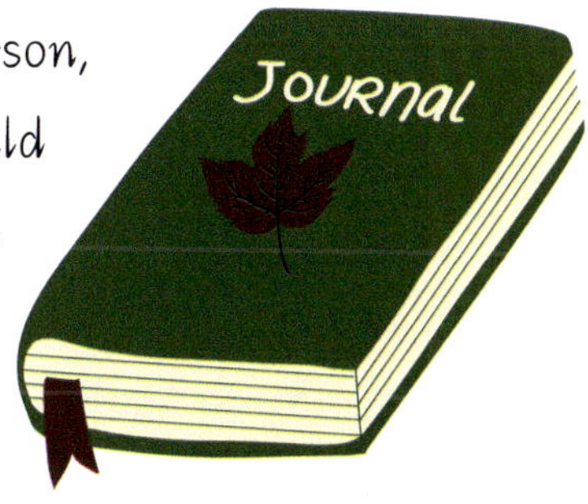

Challenging your thoughts

People often struggle to challenge their thoughts. Therefore, you might believe them even if they aren't accurate, and this can cause you additional stress and emotional instability.

When you find yourself in a thought trap, you can ask yourself how useful those thoughts are in achieving your aim. For example, if you had an exam tomorrow, and the thought - "this is not going to go well" enters your mind, would this be helpful or unhelpful?

The mind is an echo chamber, until you learn to challenge the voice inside.

You could also consider what you would say to a friend if you heard them speaking in this way. We often show others more compassion than we show ourselves.

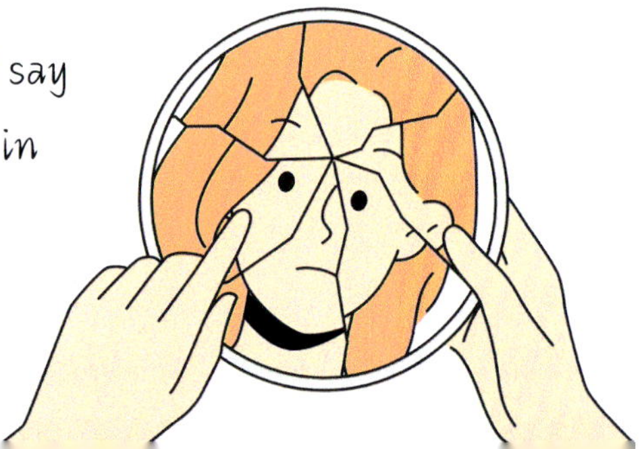

Thought challenging exercise

If you do struggle to challenge your thoughts, you could try an exercise like the one below. By keeping track of your thoughts, it becomes easier to identify when they are unhelpful. You can then practice writing a more helpful alternative, until this becomes your default.

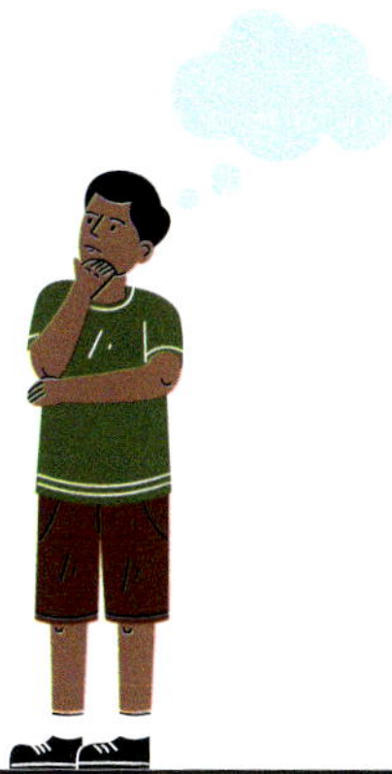

Unhelpful thoughts	Helpful alternative
"This is not going to go well"	"This might go better than I imagine"
"I have always eaten this way, I can't change"	"I have always eaten this way, but I'm open to suggestions"

Anxiety

Anxiety and stress go hand in hand. When a person is anxious, they are experiencing persistent worry, dread, and fear. This experience will cause their stress levels to rise. That is why many of the symptoms of anxiety overlap with those of stress.

Chronic anxiety also causes many of the same health issues as chronic stress. This means that a person who is chronically anxious is at higher risk of developing type 2 diabetes, cardiovascular disease, depression, and more (page 92).

My advice would be to use pages 109 and 110 to create a stress management plan which you can use when you are feeling anxious.

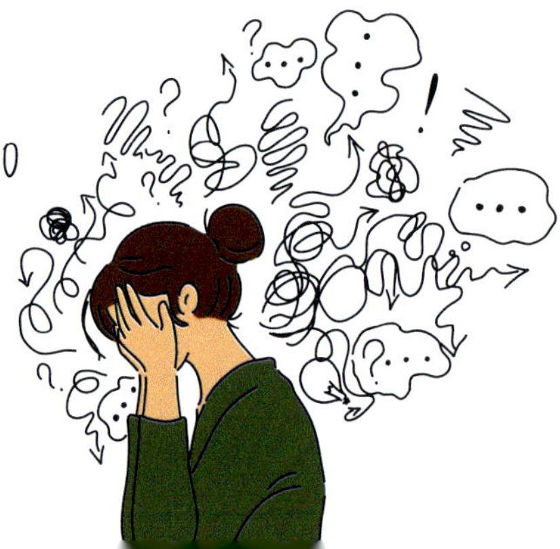

Memories can cause your stress levels to rise. For example, Post-Traumatic Stress Disorder is known as an anxiety disorder, which is caused by deeply traumatic memories that continue to affect a person after the event has passed.

In therapy, the phrase "the body keeps a score" is often used with reference to PTSD. It points to the idea that even if you try to forget or ignore a traumatic memory, the "body" remembers.

Therefore, if you ever find yourself in a similar situation to that traumatic event, or being reminded of it, you may feel your stress levels rise. The stress will prepare you to escape, because your body wants to prevent you from going through the experience again.

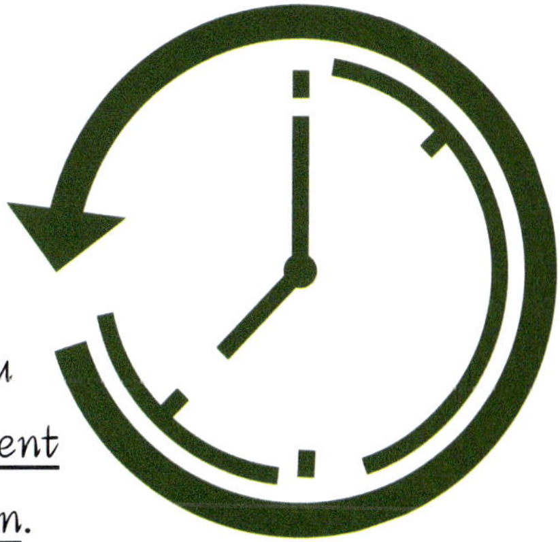

A person struggling with PTSD is likely to experience chronic stress and its associated complications, including type 2 diabetes, cardiovascular disease, and depression.

There are options available for people suffering with this disorder, including: group counselling, and Eye Movement Desensitisation Reprogramming (EMDR) therapy. The latter is a type of therapy which helps you become desensitised to traumatic memories so that your stress levels do not rise as much when you are reminded of that event.

Additionally, if you are able to develop a stress management plan, this can help reduce the impact that the traumatic memories have on you and your health.

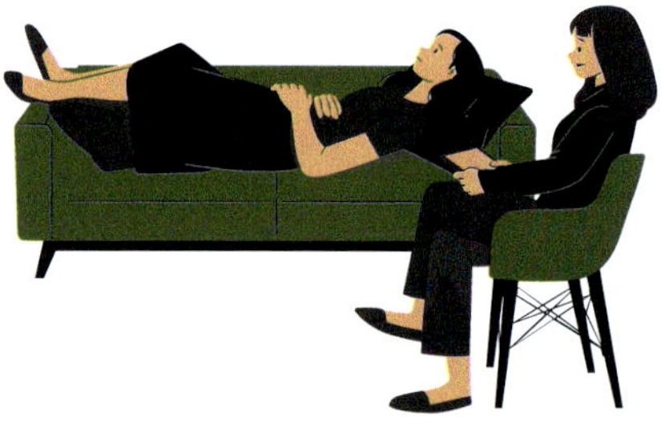

Stress related habits

People often engage in behaviours which help them deal with stress - these are stress related habits.

You might feel compelled to comfort eat, smoke a cigarette, have a glass of wine, take drugs, play games, gamble, use social media, or anything else which helps you cope. But are they really helping?

Stress related habits can be survival mechanisms. For example, when you are stressed and you crave sugary food, your body is likely craving quick-access energy, to help you survive. However, it is also because sugary foods, as well as many other behaviours and substances affect your levels of dopamine.

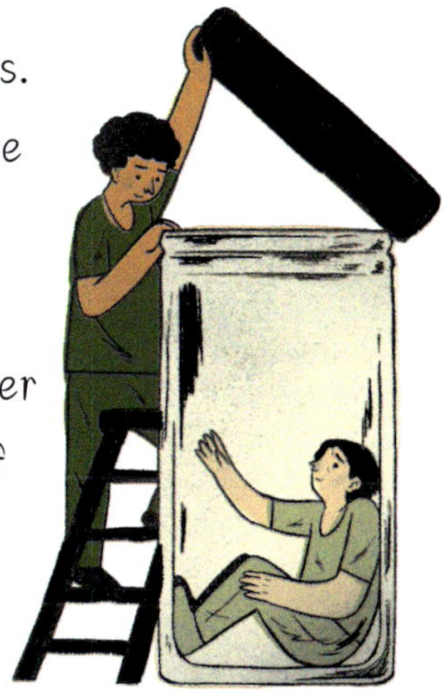

Dopamine

Dopamine is classed as a neuromodulator - this means that it can alter our brain activity. It is a chemical released from the reward centre of the brain, that helps us cope with stress, and experience pleasure, and motivation.

When we engage in certain behaviours, or consume substances that we enjoy, we have a release of dopamine. Typically, the more dopamine that is released, the more addictive that behaviour or substance becomes.

Excessive consumption of anything can be a problem. Therefore, it is important to consider how you respond to stress, and the effect that it may have on your health in the long run. Do you have any harmful habits you would like to replace or become less reliant on?

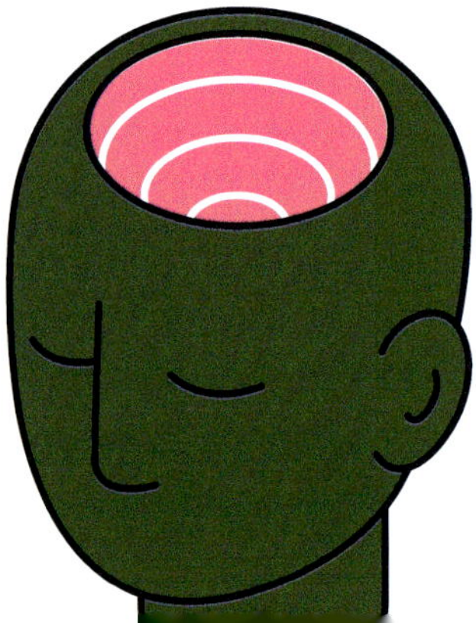

Dopamine and addiction

If a person is stressed at work, they might find that a cigarette makes them feel less stressed, in a better mood, and motivated to get back to work. Consequently, the next time they feel stressed, they are likely to repeat that cycle.

Over time, this person may require more than one cigarette to feel the same relief. This is because we become desensitised to the substances and behaviours which increase dopamine, meaning we need more. More cigarettes, food, alcohol, sex, drugs, pornography, gambling, money, social media, exercise, shopping, and any other vice.

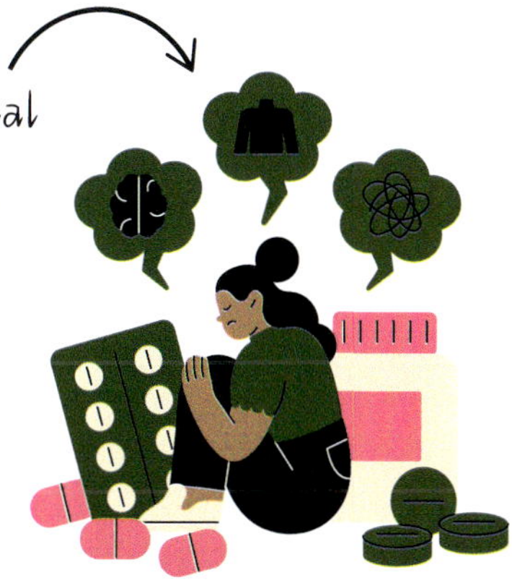

In this modern era, we excessively consume everything because it is easily accessible, and our health might be suffering as a result.

Altering habits

Understanding your habits and their long term implications can help you make more conscious decisions - because if you don't make a conscious decision, your unconscious will make it for you!

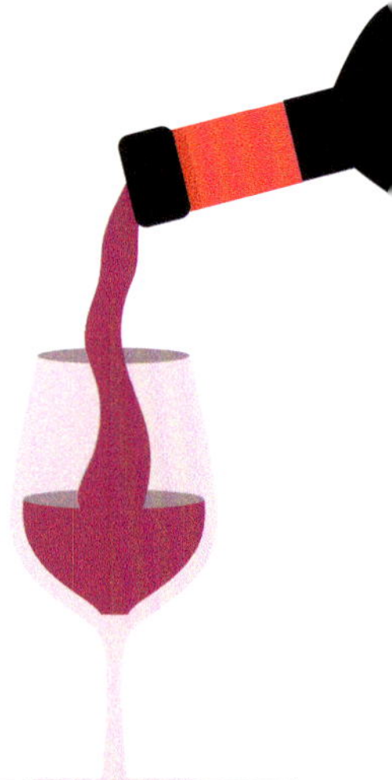

The example below highlights how you can analyse your habits and find those which could do with an adjustment. I recommend making small, simple, and enjoyable changes to your daily routines, because there are no perfect habits, just better ones.

Trigger	Routine	Reward	Implications
When I feel stressed after work	I drink a glass of wine and eat chocolate	I feel relaxed and less stressed	But I struggle to sleep at night

Stress management

So far, we have seen that stress can be due to your circumstances, thoughts, worries, anxiety, and memories. That stress can then negatively impact your health, habits, and quality of life.

Many people don't even recognise that they are stressed, because they are so fixated on the issue causing it. However, prolonged periods of stress WILL have a negative effect on your health. Therefore, it is important to practice managing your stress better, regardless of the situation.

I believe it is important for everybody to have a stress management plan. It may not eradicate stress from your life, but it can help you to recognise stress sooner and respond to it in a healthier way.

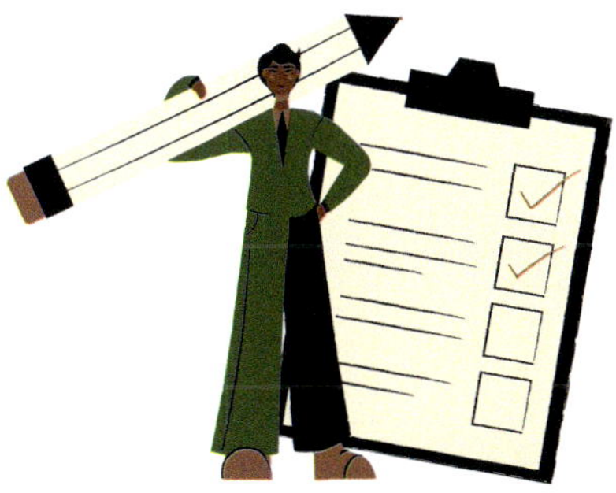

Stress management plan template

The structure below can help you create your own stress management plan. Columns 1 and 2 are for identifying stress, and column 3 is for taking action to reduce that stress.

I recommend inputting as many answers as you can, making it unique to you, and leaving it somewhere you will see it, like the fridge!

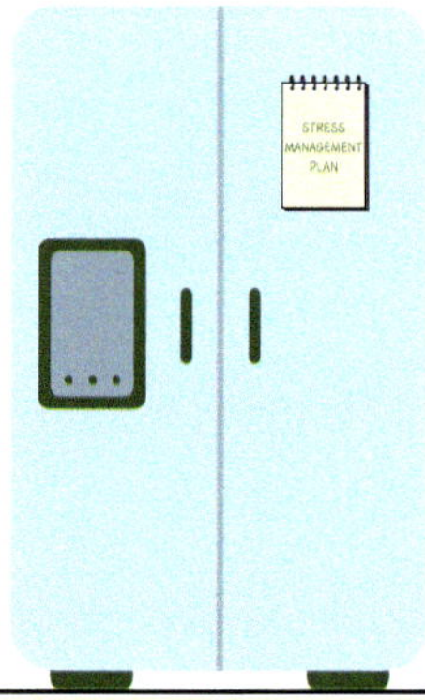

(1) What are my stress symptoms?	(2) What are my stress-related habits?	(3) What activities help me de-stress?
Heavy breathing	Drinking wine	Journalling
Anger	Eating chocolate	Yoga
Sweating		Breathing exercises

Stress relieving activities

Below is a list of stress relieving activities for your plan. The benefit of including more than one, is that you can combine them, or perform them sequentially, making them more effective.

Breathing exercises	Reading a book
Going for a walk	Exercising + stretching
Cooking + baking	Cleaning + organising
Listening to music	Creative activities
Yoga + meditation	Puzzles + games
Speaking to a friend	Writing in a journal
Thinking out loud	Knitting + crocheting

Which ones can you add to your plan?

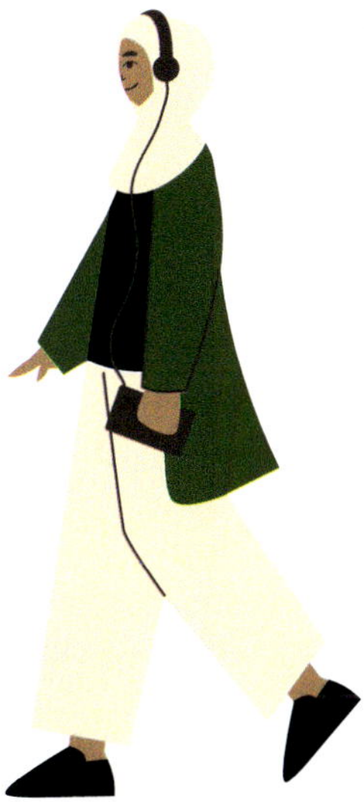

Reflection point 4

This is a list of suggestions based on the information from this section:

- Understand the effect of stress on your health and recognise your stress symptoms.
- Notice what is causing you stress (your circumstances, thoughts, perceptions, worries, memories...).
- Understand and look out for the connection between anxiety and stress.
- Practice challenging your thoughts and getting out of your head with the methods listed in this section.
- Become aware of your stress-related habits.
- Use the template to produce your own stress management plan.
- Keep the plan somewhere you can see it.

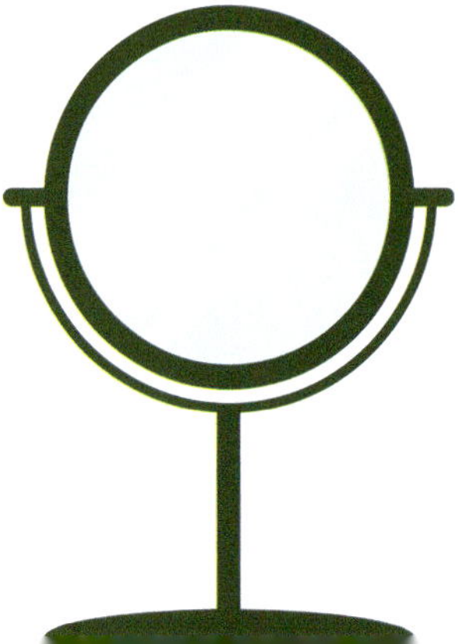

Section 5
THE IMPORTANCE OF SLEEP

"Sleep is the golden chain that ties health and our bodies together."

— Thomas Dekker

Sleep

Sleep is very important for almost every living creature on earth - particularly humans. Sleep enables the brain and body to undergo the repair and restoration that is required for us to function correctly and remain in good health.

Sleep deprivation, on the other hand, is linked with type 2 diabetes, cardiovascular disease, high blood pressure, obesity, depression, anxiety, dementia, kidney disease, inflammation, and oxidative stress. It is a very important topic.

Your ability to sleep is affected by many of the topics that we have already explored in this guide, and there are plenty of other factors to be aware of. For that reason, it is again important to be holistic and make small changes where possible.

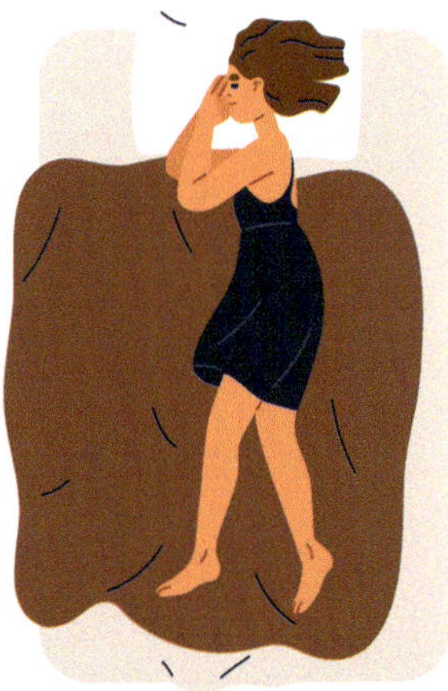

Sleep and diabetes

When your blood sugar levels are high, the body gets rid of the excess sugar by urinating it out (page 2). For this reason, when your blood sugar levels are elevated at night, you are likely to wake up more frequently to go to the toilet.

If this is continuous and disrupts your ability to sleep, you may become sleep deprived. Sleep deprivation can cause your body to produce less insulin.

If your body produces less insulin, over time your blood sugar will become even more unstable, potentially making you wake up more frequently, leading to yet more sleep deprivation. This cycle then repeats. To add to this issue, people often crave sugary foods when they are sleep deprived.

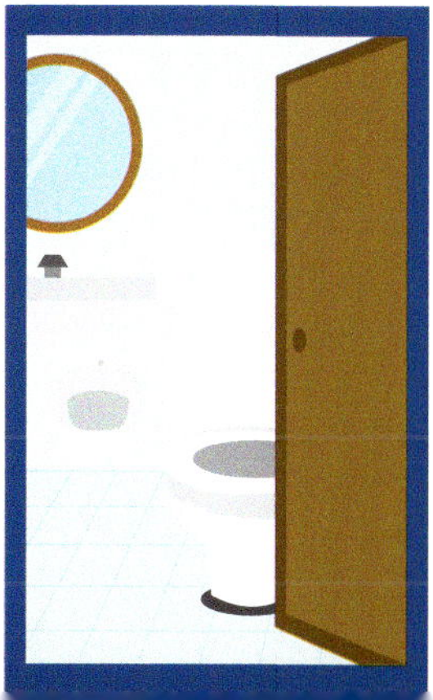

Sleep-wake cycle

The hormones, cortisol and melatonin, control the sleep-wake cycle.

Cortisol, one of the stress hormones mentioned on page 91, is responsible for waking you up in the morning, by causing your blood sugar to rise. This hormone is produced by the adrenal glands.

Melatonin, on the other hand, helps you fall asleep and is produced by an area of the brain called the Pineal Gland.

If your cortisol levels are high, and melatonin levels are low, this can prevent you from falling asleep. Therefore, it is important to understand the factors which affect these hormones and make the necessary adjustments.

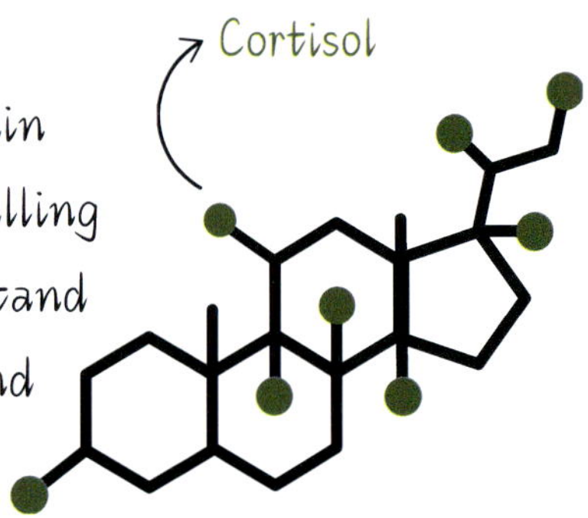

Circadian rhythms

Circadian rhythms are natural bodily cycles that repeat every 24 hours. This is the body clock.

These cycles dictate the automatic changes that take place in the brain and body, every day and night. They regulate bodily functions such as: blood sugar, appetite, and sleep - by influencing the production of cortisol and melatonin.

There are many factors which affect your circadian rhythms, such as: your sleep routine, activity levels, light exposure, nutrition, and stress, among others. Taking control of these factors, and forming healthy and consistent routines, can help you improve the way your body regulates itself automatically. Sleep is just one part of that puzzle.

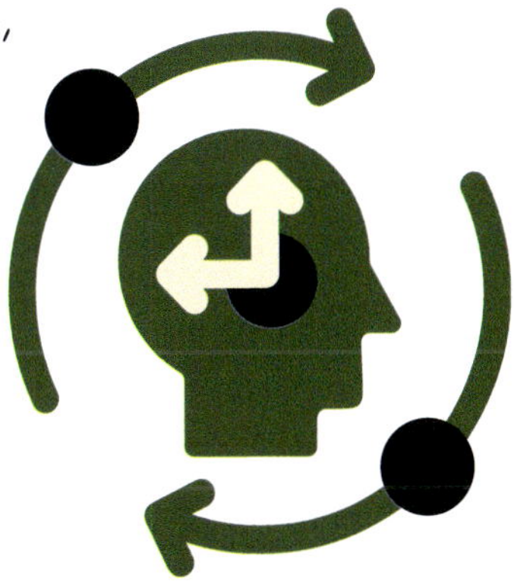

Sleep stages

Throughout the night, you go through multiple stages of sleep which allow for the restoration of your brain and body, and consolidation of memory and information. The sleep stages are as follows:

1. Non-REM 1 (the lightest and shortest stage)
2. Non-REM 2 (the longest stage)
3. Non-REM 3 (the deepest and most restorative stage)
4. REM (the stage in which you are most likely to experience vivid dreams and paralysis to prevent you from acting out the dreams)

A sleep cycle involves completing every sleep stage, and takes around 90 minutes. To get enough deep rest, adults need to complete around five sleep cycles per night, which equates to 7.5 hours of sleep.

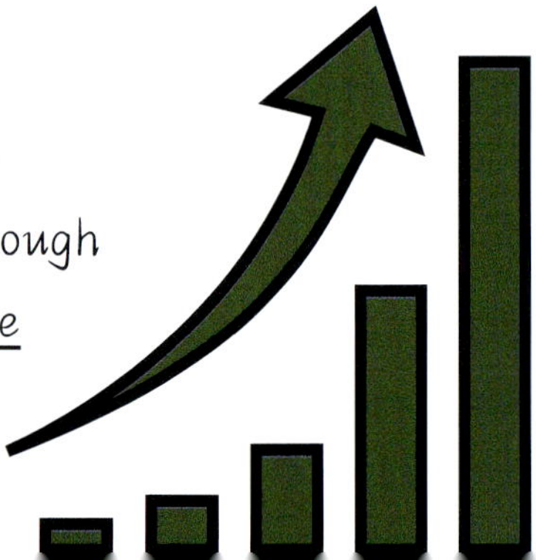

Sleep guidance

Throughout the rest of this section, I will suggest methods of improving your sleep. They may not all work for you, but even a slight improvement can dramatically improve your health.

I would suggest keeping a sleep diary to assess how different behaviours affect your sleep. The example below may make a useful guide.

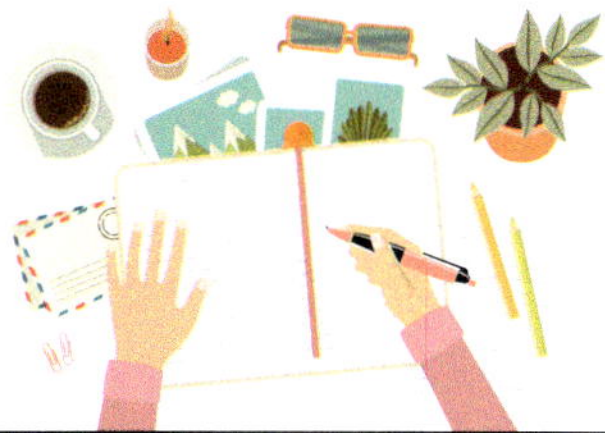

Date	Behaviour before bed	Bedtime	Sleep quality (/10)	Sleep duration (hours)
17/12/24	Reading a book	10pm	8	7.5
18/12/24	Scrolling social media	1am	4	5

Routine and timing

How many times do you fall asleep in front of the tv, and feel wide awake by the time you go to bed? This is because tiredness comes in waves, and if you miss the boat, you might have to wait for the next wave.

It is important to develop a routine that revolves around the optimal time for you to fall asleep. For example, if you know that 11pm is when you are most likely to fall asleep, arranging your routine so that you are in bed by that time every day is key to avoid missing the boat and improving your circadian rhythms.

Furthermore, your body and brain thrive on routine. The longer you maintain it, the more effective they will become in the long run.

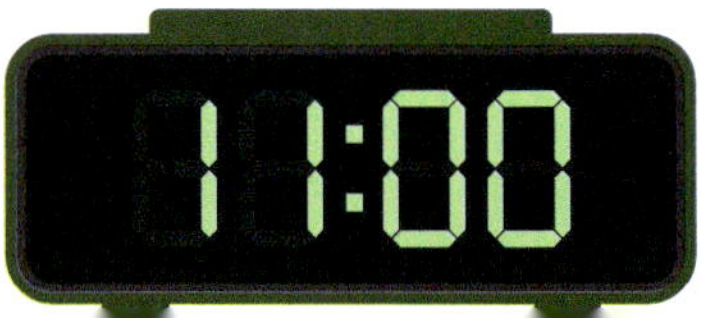

Blood sugar

As mentioned on page 113, when your blood sugar levels are high, you are likely to get up more frequently to go to the toilet in the night. To counter this, you could consider making changes to your diet and activity levels.

For starters, you could stop eating, or eat less, 1 to 4 hours before going to bed. This allows time for your blood sugar to return to normal before you fall asleep.

You could also turn back to the glycemic index section (page 26), to adjust your food choices and preparation. Additionally, you could consume more foods and drinks that contain antioxidants (page 46) to improve your body's response to insulin.

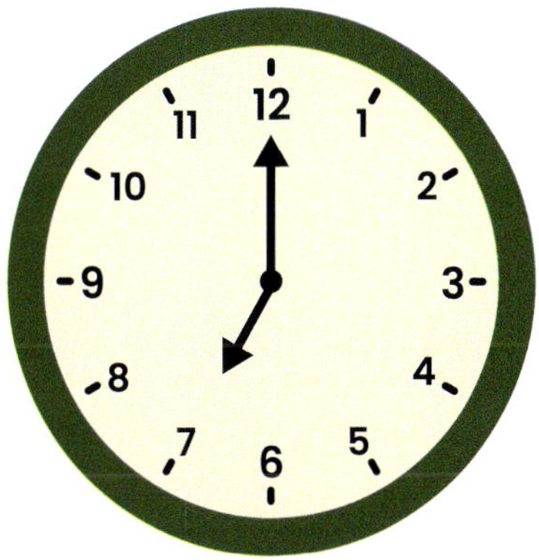

Blood sugar

It is important to consider that all exercise is useful and beneficial. However, as I mention on page 76, exercising at high intensities will likely cause your blood sugar to rise temporarily. As a result, exercising at high intensities in the evening/night can negatively impact sleep.

I would suggest doing high intensity exercise earlier in the day, so that you have time to allow your blood sugar to return to normal before bed.

I also recommend doing low intensity exercise at any time, but if it's done later in the day, this can be particularly useful for controlling your blood sugar. Some people walk their dog after dinner, or do light chair exercises while they watch the tv.

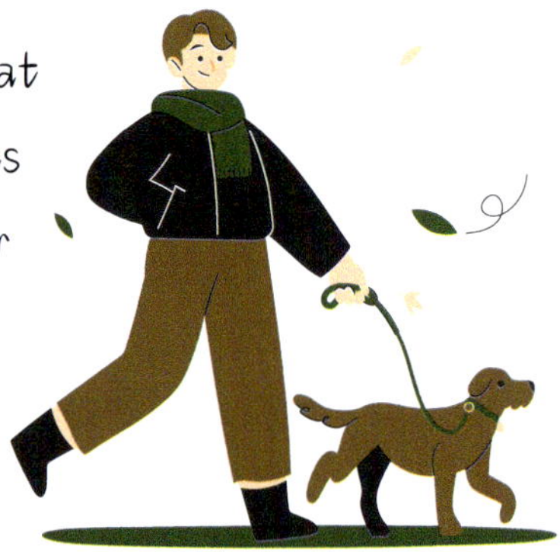

Naps

Research shows that napping can improve elements of your physical and mental state, including: your memory, ability to learn, stress levels, blood pressure, immune system, and athletic performance.

Napping has been practiced for generations by numerous cultures. The prophet Muhammad called the midday nap 'qailulah', and the word 'siesta' is a latin phrase still used today to describe an afternoon nap. This is practiced by many cultures, particularly those living in warm climates.

Napping may or may not work for you as an individual, but they are shown to help people get more rest day to day. 20 minutes at 2pm is meant to be the optimal nap for most people.

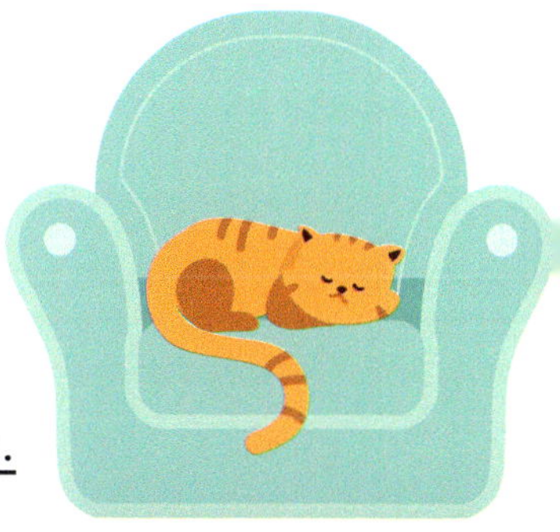

Light

Melatonin is a hormone which is produced by the Pineal gland and helps you fall asleep (page 114). Certain forms of light, such as: sunlight, LED bulbs, LED screens, and florescent light, can disrupt the pineal gland and prevent it from producing as much melatonin. Potentially preventing you from falling asleep. This is because they are 'blue lights', which operate at a high frequency.

To reduce the amount of blue light your eyes are exposed to, you could use a dim lamp or a sleep light. You could also use blue light lenses, switch on 'night mode' on your devices, and reduce your overall screen time. If you practice these changes later in the day, you may find that getting to sleep is easier.

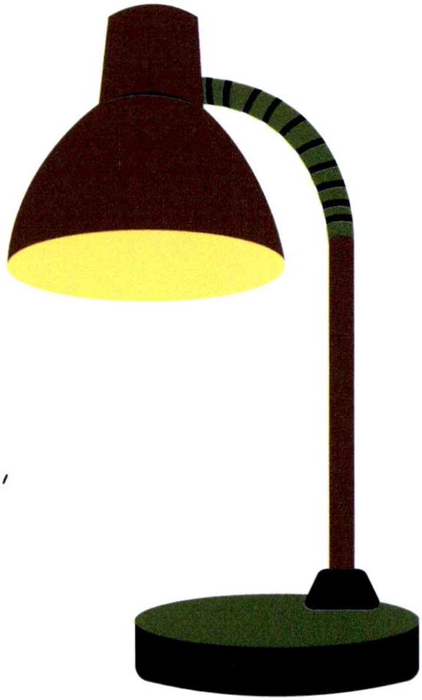

Temperature

As bedtime approaches, your internal temperature should begin to fall by 1 - 2° C. This is an example of a circadian rhythm (page 116). Therefore, the optimal temperature for falling asleep is between 18°C and 20°C (65-68°F). This is the reason you are likely to sleep better in the winter as opposed to the summer.

However, some people prefer a warmer environment. It is worth trialing different temperatures to see what works best for you.

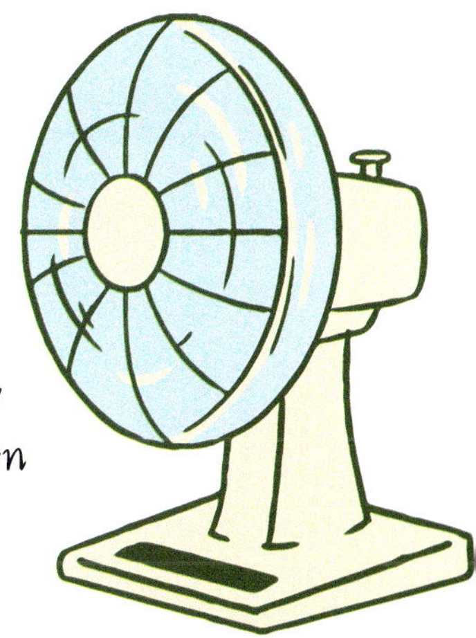

To reduce the temperature, you could sleep with thinner clothing, use a fan, or adjust the heat settings in your house. Alternatively, a hot shower or bath can actually cool you down because when your skin is warm, your internal temperature decreases to compensate.

Sound

Experimenting with sound, by either adding it or taking it away, can also help improve your sleep.

Some people need complete silence to sleep. If that is the case for yourself, you could try using ear plugs or noise cancelling ear or headphones.

Other people prefer having background noise. You could put on an audiobook or podcast with a timer so that it turns off after a specified duration. You could follow a guided meditation, or use a sleep sounds app so that you can listen to white noise, rain, or any other sounds that relax you. Alternatively, the suggestion about using a fan could help you cool your room and introduce some background noise at the same time.

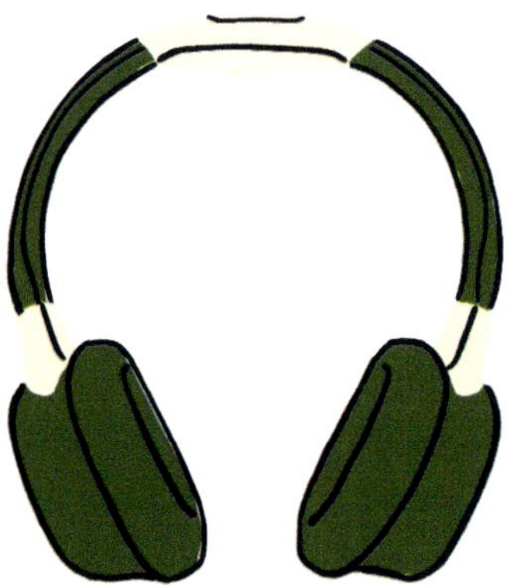

Stress and thoughts

How many times have you been awake for hours due to your thoughts, stress, and worries?

If for example, you find yourself catastrophising at night (page 97), you are likely to begin to feel stressed, which can prevent you from falling asleep. Stress increases your cortisol and blood sugar levels, makes you more alert, and prepares your brain and body for action, even if it isn't required. This is not a conducive state for falling asleep.

This further highlights the importance of developing a stress management plan (page 109). If you are able to create a routine that helps you de-stress, this can help you fall asleep. My personal plan involves journalling, reading, and breathing exercises.

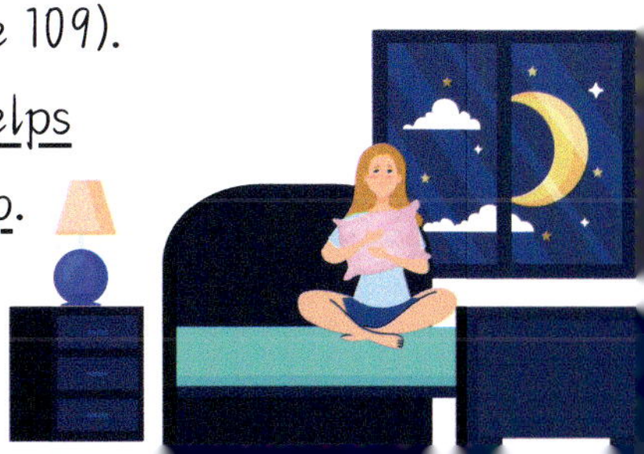

Breathing exercises

Breath control is taught to soldiers, fire fighters, martial artists, athletes, police officers, and anybody else who requires control over their physical and mental state. Controlled breathing can help you to change how you are feeling in this very moment, but they require practice.

Breathing exercises are incredibly useful for reducing your stress levels and falling asleep.

Slow breathing, particularly in and out through the nose, can reduce your adrenaline and cortisol levels (page 114), heart rate, breathing rate, and blood pressure. If you do them for long enough, they can indirectly help you to control your blood sugar, by reducing your stress levels and getting more sleep.

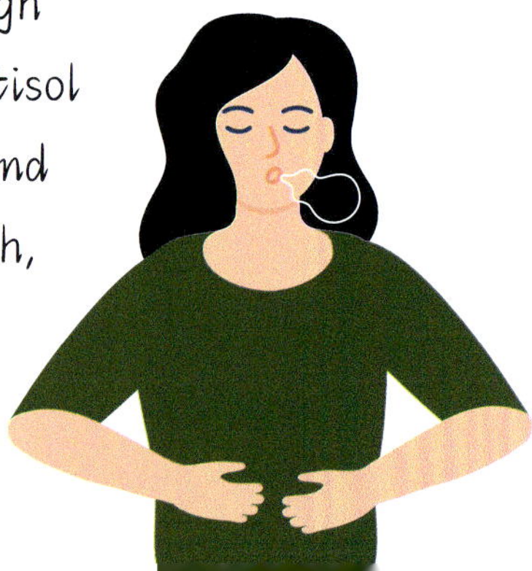

Triangle and square breathing 127

In my experience, breathing exercises which you can visualise are useful tools, and can help you avoid getting distracted.

Below are two you could try for yourself. For both of them, attempt to follow each side of the shape for 4 seconds (e.g. inhale for 4 → hold for 4 → exhale for 4).

Some people prefer holding for longer or shorter durations, so you could try 3 seconds or 5 seconds. Just remember to only do what feels comfortable.

Breathing exercises are often taught at yoga, meditation, and mindfulness classes and there are plenty of other exercises you can learn.

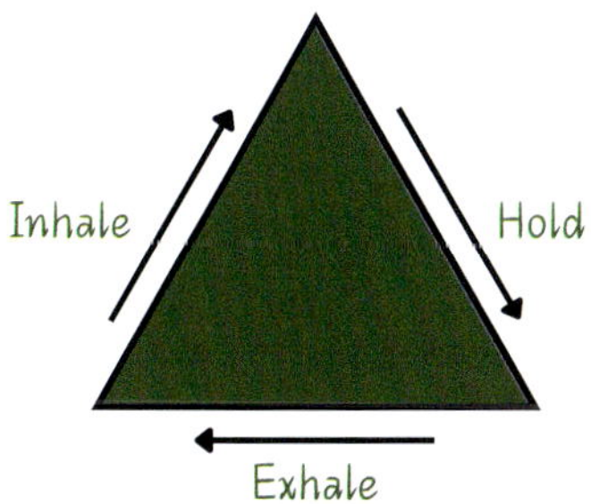

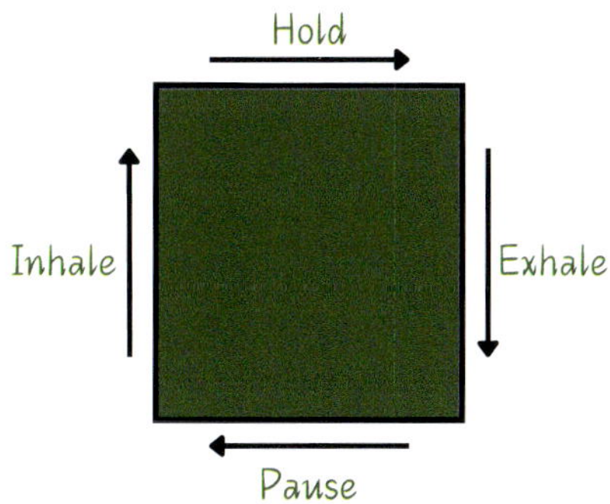

Waking up guide

If you want to feel more alert in the morning, you could consider altering your waking routine.

Exposing your eyes to direct sunlight in the morning can help you wake up easier because it causes your cortisol levels to rise. That does not mean looking directly at the sun, but rather being outside, instead of looking through glass.

Additionally, physical activity can have the same effect. Therefore, you could combine the two and go for a walk in the morning.

Finally, waking up at a similar time everyday can improve your circadian rhythms. This means that waking up may get easier, as well as falling asleep.

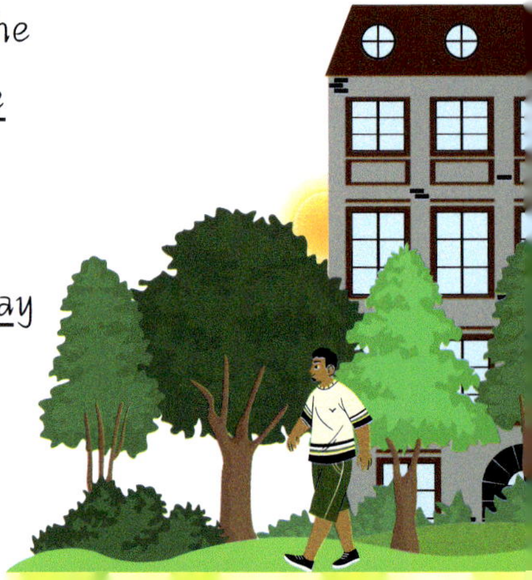

Caffeine alone does not have a direct effect on blood sugar. However, it does connect to the topics of sleep, stress, and nutrition.

Caffeine is a stimulant that increases feelings of alertness and focus, and reduces feelings of tiredness. For this reason, caffeine can have a negative effect on your ability to sleep. Reducing your consumption of caffeine anytime after midday is generally recommended if you struggle with sleep.

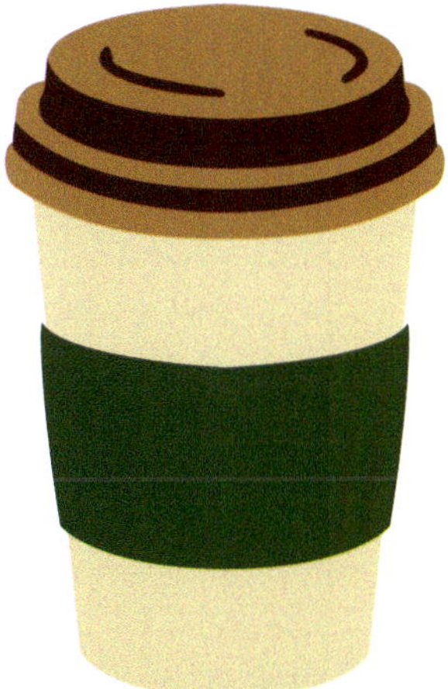

Additionally, caffeine can increase your adrenaline and cortisol levels, and therefore your stress levels, especially if consumed while you are already stressed. This can result in an increase in blood sugar.

Caffeinated drinks

Caffeine is often found in drinks like coffee, tea, energy drinks and pre-workout shakes - all of which may also have added sugar. This is just something to be aware of, especially considering how many caffeinated drinks you may consume on a daily basis.

Overall, caffeine consumption does not have a direct effect on your risk of developing type 2 diabetes, but it can have an indirect effect.

If you would like to improve your relationship with caffeine, I would suggest taking note of how frequently you consume caffeinated drinks, the content of sugar inside of them, the effect that they have on your stress levels, and how they impact your sleep patterns.

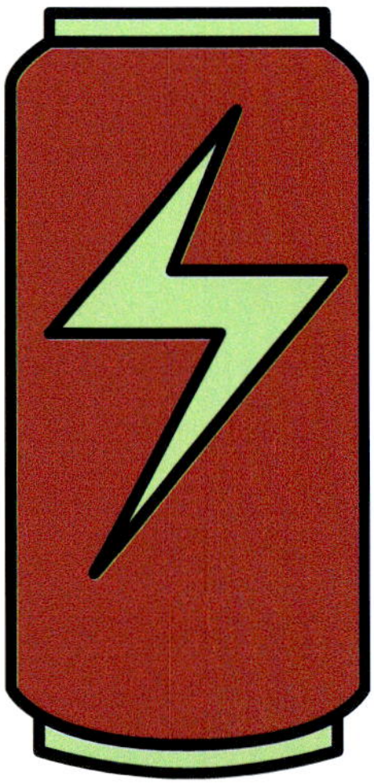

Alcohol overview

When it comes to alcohol, it is all about moderation, because long term and excessive consumption of any alcohol can increase your risk of cardiovascular disease, liver disease, and dementia.

Excessive drinking can also increase insulin resistance, putting you at greater risk of developing type 2 diabetes. Therefore, it is recommended by the NHS that you don't drink more than 14 units per week, ideally spread across at least 3 days or more.

14 units is equivalent to 6 medium glasses of wine, 6 pints of beer, 5 ciders, OR 14 shots. There are alcohol support links towards the end of the book if you feel like you might need help.

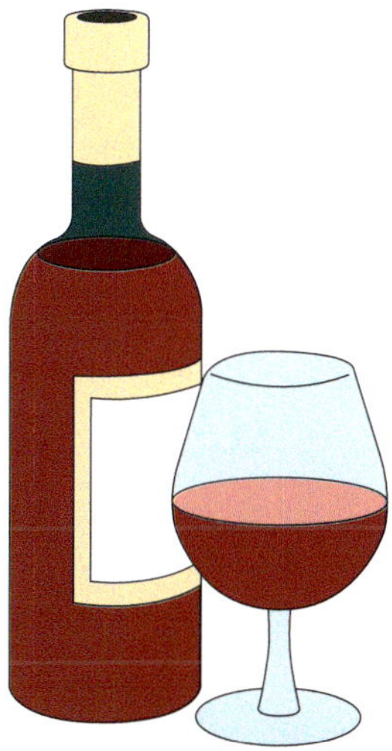

Alcohol and stress

Alcohol can increase your stress hormones: cortisol and adrenaline, meaning that although alcohol might temporarily make you feel better when you are stressed or anxious, in the long run it is likely to make matters worse.

The reason why alcohol makes you feel better is partly because you experience a rise in your dopamine levels. As mentioned on page 105, dopamine helps lift your mood, makes you feel motivated, and reduces your stress levels.

However, over time, you will likely need more alcohol to get the desired effect, which is why people often become reliant on alcohol, as the image to the right demonstrates.

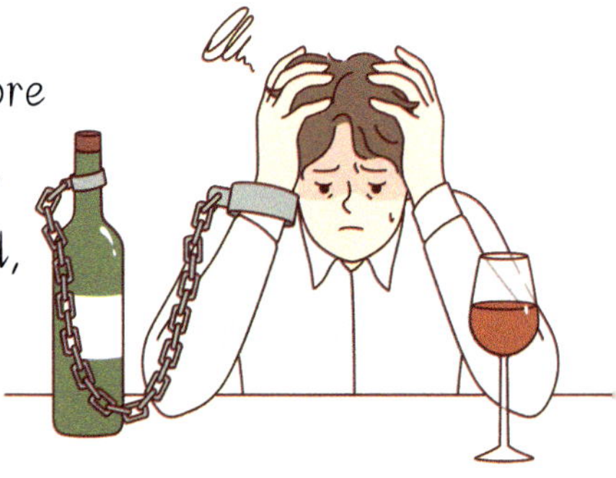

Alcohol and sleep

Alcohol can negatively impact your ability to get into the deeper stages of sleep, and makes you more likely to wake up during the night. This can lead to sleep deprivation, and your body producing less insulin. This is explained further on page 113.

In the long run, alcohol can severely disrupt your sleep patterns and circadian rhythms. As a result, you are likely to feel worse over time, and experience the negative consequences of both consistent alcohol use and sleep deprivation.

Therefore, it is important to consider your alcohol use, and begin making reductions where possible. Even a slight change can yield positive results for your health.

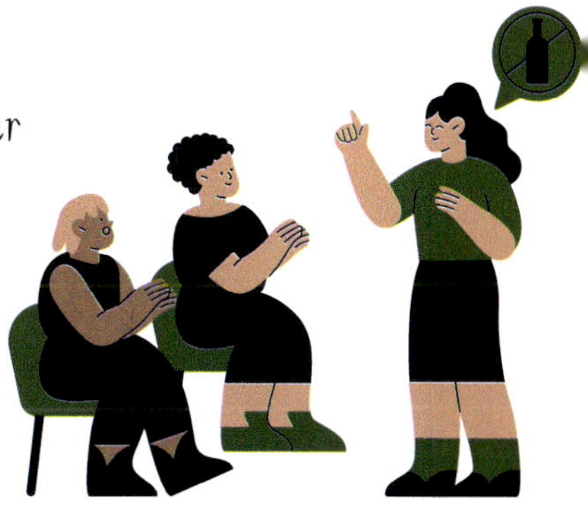

Nicotine overview

Nicotine can make you feel more alert, improve memory, and increase levels of dopamine in your brain. This can explain why it often helps people feel more focussed and less stressed - but it is also, in part, why nicotine is so addictive.

Globally, nicotine, from tobacco products in particular, are known to cause around 8 million deaths per year, and an additional 1.3 million deaths due to second-hand smoke inhalation. Many of these deaths would have been caused by cardiovascular disease, respiratory disorders, and cancer, as a result of smoking.

As well as being harmful for the reasons listed above, nicotine is also linked to a greater risk of type 2 diabetes.

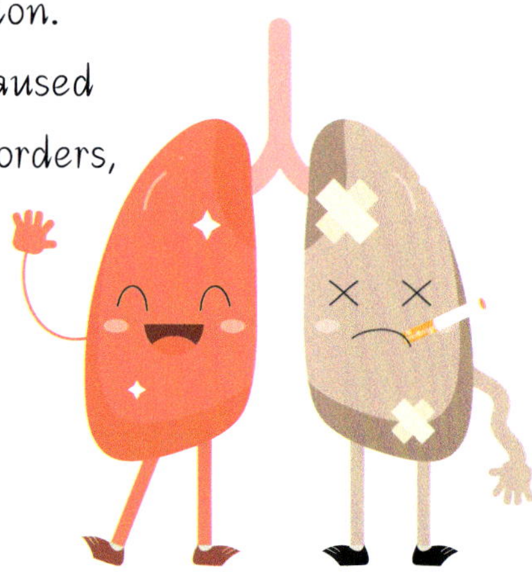

Nicotine, stress, and sleep

All nicotine-containing products can affect the way the body's cells respond to insulin - potentially leading to insulin resistance.

Additionally, nicotine stimulates the body to release more cortisol and adrenaline, meaning that it can also increase your stress levels, and therefore, cause a rise in blood sugar (page 91).

Furthermore, nicotine is associated with higher rates of insomnia and sleep apnoea - leading to sleep deprivation, which can lead to the body producing less insulin over time (page 113).

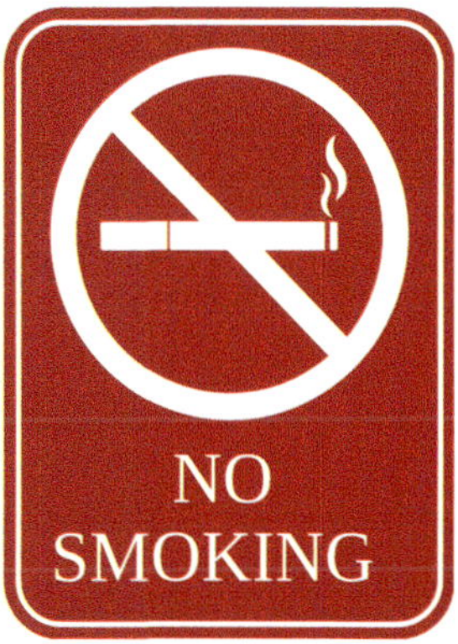

Overall, smoking can greatly increase your risk of type 2 diabetes. For this reason, there are links at the end of the book which can offer you support.

Medication

Certain medications can cause your blood sugar to rise and increase the risk of developing type 2 diabetes. Such medications include beta-blockers, thiazide diuretics, anti-psychotics, cholesterol medication, and certain antidepressants.

Statins, for example, are a commonly prescribed form of medication which helps people control their cholesterol levels, and their risk of cardio-vascular disease. As effective and necessary as they are, research has shown that they can lead to an increase in blood sugar.

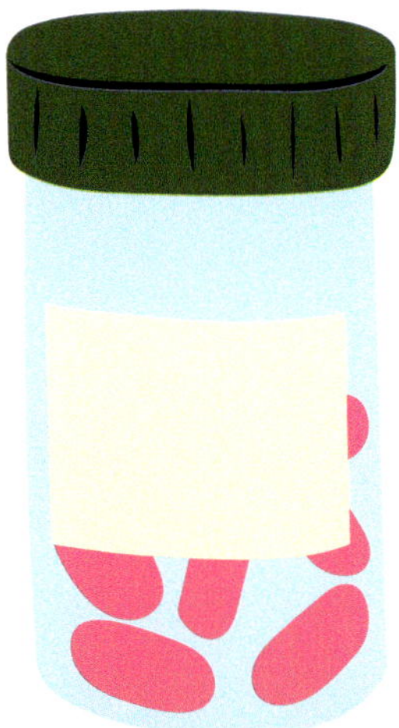

This does not guarantee that your medication is causing your blood sugar to rise, but it is a possibility. However, DO NOT adjust your medication without consulting your GP.

Medication and sleep

Many prescription and over-the-counter medications, including antidepressants, decongestants, steroids, statins, diuretics, and even sleep medications <u>can cause sleep disruption</u>. If taken continuously, this can contribute to sleep deprivation (page 112).

For medications like statins, which can cause a rise in blood sugar <u>and</u> difficulty sleeping, I often recommend taking them earlier in the day - <u>but you must discuss with your GP first</u>.

By taking them earlier, you'll have time in the day to <u>reduce your blood sugar by night</u>, which will hopefully improve your ability to sleep, and reduce the risk of type 2 diabetes.

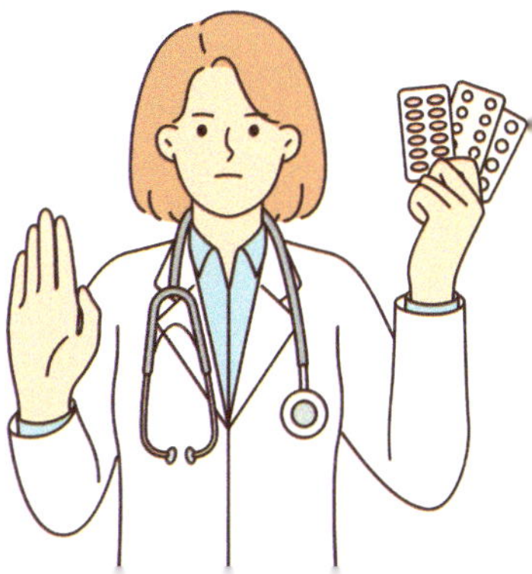

Reflection point 5

This is a list of suggestions based on the information from this section:

- Create a sleep diary and begin trialling new methods of falling asleep to see what works and what doesn't.
- Create a nightly routine and bedtime.
- Eat lower GI foods, adjust the GI of the foods you eat, and do light exercise to control your blood sugar before going to bed.
- Consider environmental factors like light, sound, noise, and temperature.
- Use your stress management plan when stress is keeping you up at night.
- Go for a walk outside in the morning.
- Consider your use of nicotine, alcohol, caffeine, and medication in relation to sleep.

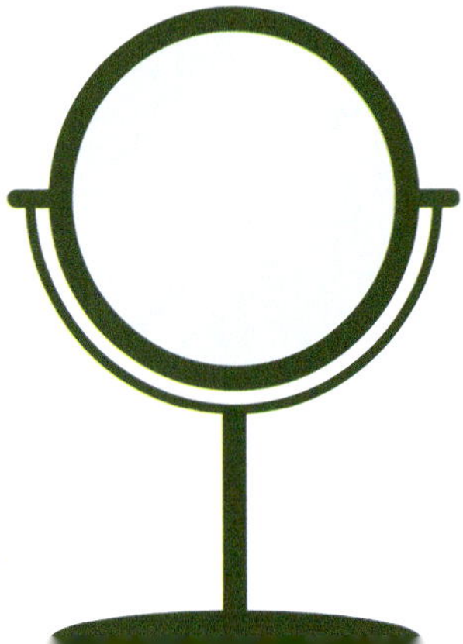

Section 6
CONNECTING HEALTH ISSUES

"To keep the body in good health is a duty, otherwise we shall not be able to keep our mind strong and clear."

— Buddha

Connecting health issues

So far, I have demonstrated that your health is affected by many factors, and we have explored topics like nutrition, physical activity, stress, sleep, bodyweight, and our daily habits.

All of the topics mentioned so far link to type 2 diabetes in one way or another, but they also apply to a number of other health conditions, which we will explore in the upcoming pages.

The purpose of this section is to demonstrate how interconnected your health is, and why taking small steps to improve one issue can benefit you in multiple ways. For example, by managing your risk of type 2 diabetes, you can also reduce the risk and severity of conditions like cardiovascular disease!

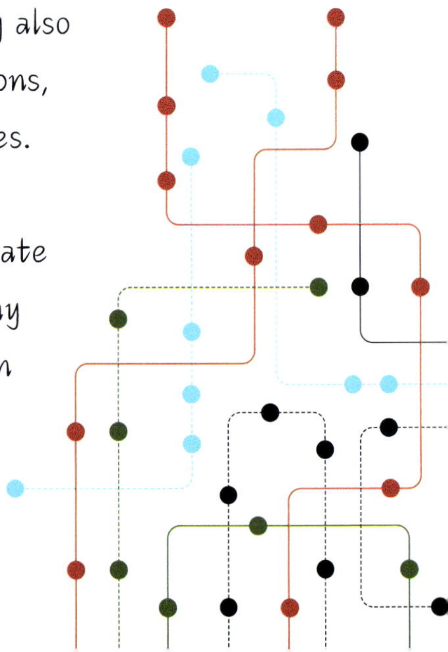

Inflammation

Inflammation is the body's way of defending against pathogens, injuries, and illness, and can occur across the entire body, or in localised areas.

Acute inflammation can occur for minutes, hours, days, and possibly weeks, and is usually accompanied by redness, heat, swelling, and/or pain. Examples include: the redness, swelling, and heat around a fresh wound, or the fever you develop when you have the flu.

Chronic inflammation however can last for weeks, months, and even years. Chronic inflammation is associated with type 2 diabetes, cardiovascular disease, oxidative stress, depression, anxiety, arthritis, Alzheimer's, Crohn's disease, asthma, fatigue, COPD, autoimmune disorders, and a weakened immune system.

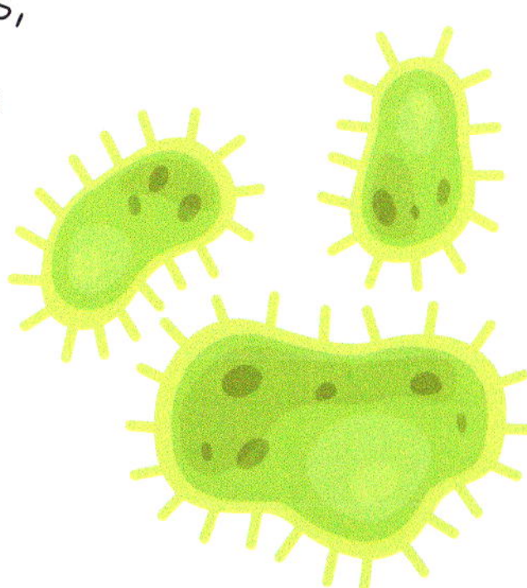

Causes of inflammation

The factors listed below can all lead to elevated levels of inflammation around the body. By making lifestyle adjustments, you can reduce your levels of inflammation and avoid it becoming chronic.

- Processed foods
- Excessive salt intake
- Fried foods
- Trans fats
- Low levels of activity
- Chronic stress
- Having excess body fat
- Sleep deprivation
- Toxins (e.g. air pollution)
- Tobacco products
- Excessive alcohol intake
- Poor gut health

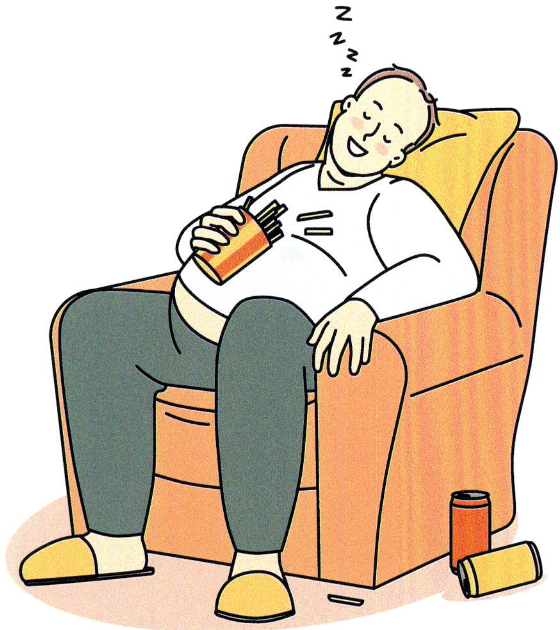

Reducing inflammation

Addressing the factors mentioned on the previous page can be a good step towards reducing your levels of inflammation. Additionally, including these anti-inflammatory foods and drinks in your diet can help as well:

Berries and citrus fruits	Spinach, kale, garlic, and onions
Salmon, mackerel, tuna, and sardines	Turmeric, black pepper, ginger, and cinnamon
Avocados, avocado oil, and olive oil	Almonds, cashews, and sesame seeds
Antioxidant rich food (page 46)	Probiotic rich food (page 147)

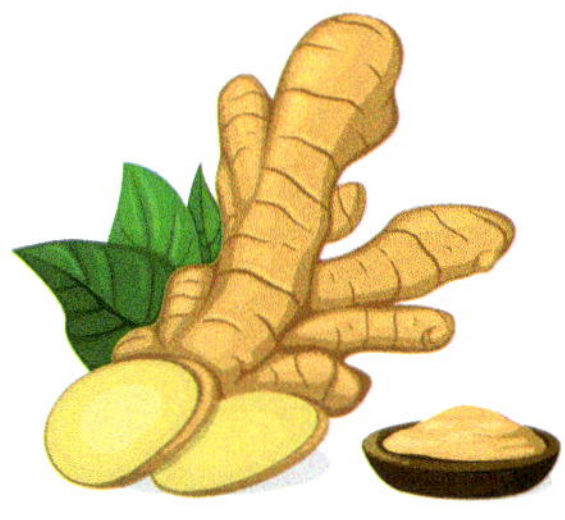

Oxidative stress

Inside of your body are little molecules called 'free radicals', these are waste products which are harmful if too many accumulate in the body.

Free radicals are harmful because, at an atomic level, they are missing an electron, which makes them unstable. Therefore, when free radicals travel around the body, they steal the electrons they find, thus damaging cells, proteins, and even DNA. This damage is known as 'oxidative stress'.

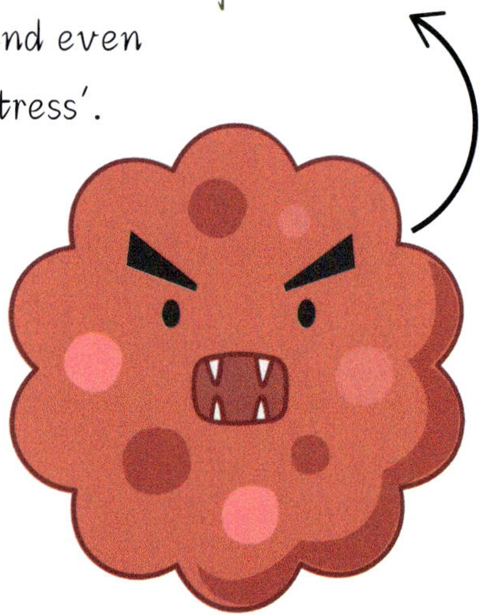

To combat this issue, antioxidants will neutralise a free radical by sharing an electron, so that they don't take them from your body. Eating more antioxidant rich foods can reduce your levels of oxidative stress (page 46).

Oxidative stress

As a result of the damage mentioned on the previous page, oxidative stress can lead to many health complications, including: type 2 diabetes, cardiovascular disease, lung disease, kidney disease, depression, and neurological diseases like Alzheimer's and Parkinson's. It is a major problem.

Oxidative stress is another issue which connects all of the topics in this book. It can be caused by: processed foods, excessive amounts of unhealthy fat and sugar, lack of exercise, too much exercise, lack of sleep, chronic stress, tobacco, alcohol, and inflammation.

I recommend using this book to add balance to these areas of your health, bit by bit, to reduce your levels of oxidative stress.

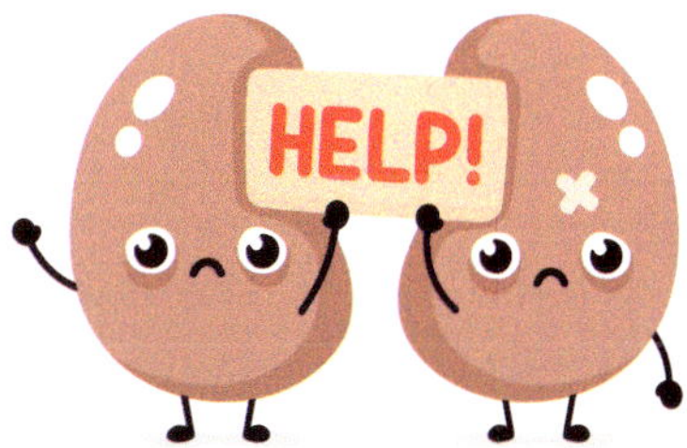

Gut health

The gut includes your stomach, intestines and colon, and inside is your gut microbiome. The microbiome contains bacteria, viruses, and fungi. Collectively, they live as part of an ecosystem inside of you, that is affected by how you live your life and what you put into your body. This ecosystem is important for digestion, metabolism, hunger, immunity, and hormone production.

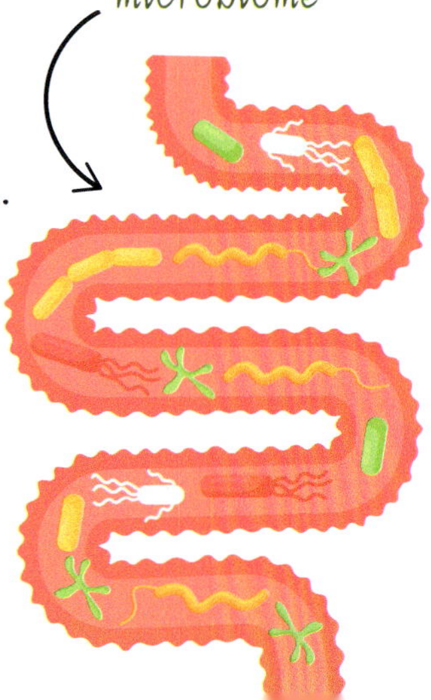

Research indicates that diversity in the gut is one of the most important factors for gut health. This means your microbiome should contain a large variety of microbes. If a person lacks diversity in their gut, they are at greater risk of developing conditions like type 2 diabetes, cardiovascular disease, liver disease, depression, digestive disorders, and inflammation.

Gut-brain axis

The 'gut-brain axis' is a term used to describe the reciprocal relationship between the gut and the brain. More information is transferred between the two than anywhere else in the body.

Second to the brain, the gut also contains more nerves than any other area of the body, and is commonly known as the 'second brain'.

Because of the gut-brain connection, the health of your gut influences your physical and mental health. Levels of depression, anxiety, stress, and overall cognition are affected by how well the gut metabolises food, and communicates with the immune, and nervous systems. Therefore, it is important to maintain a healthy gut.

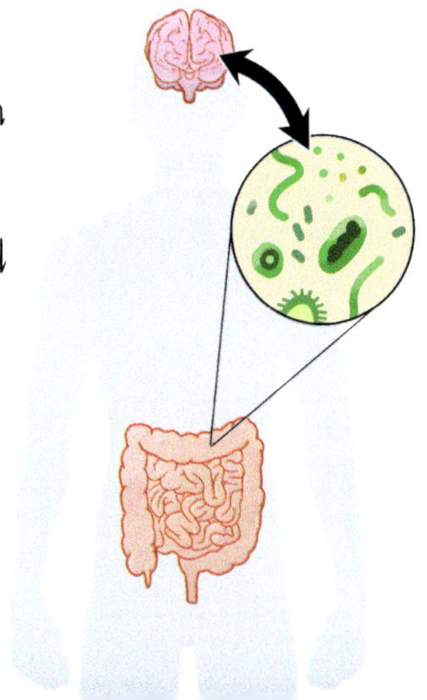

Improving gut health

To improve your gut health, you can start by increasing your activity levels, reducing your stress levels, eating plenty of fibre, and including some of these foods in your diet:

Probiotics	Prebiotics
• Yoghurt (especially with 'live cultures') • Kefir • Kimchi • Sauerkraut • Tempeh • Miso • Kombucha • Pickles (that have not been pasteurised and are made with salt, not vinegar)	• Asparagus • Garlic • Onion • Banana • Chicory • Raw honey • Soybean • Barley • Almonds • Pulses • Jerusalem artichoke

Probiotics introduce new microbes to the gut!

Prebiotics are food for the microbes in the gut!

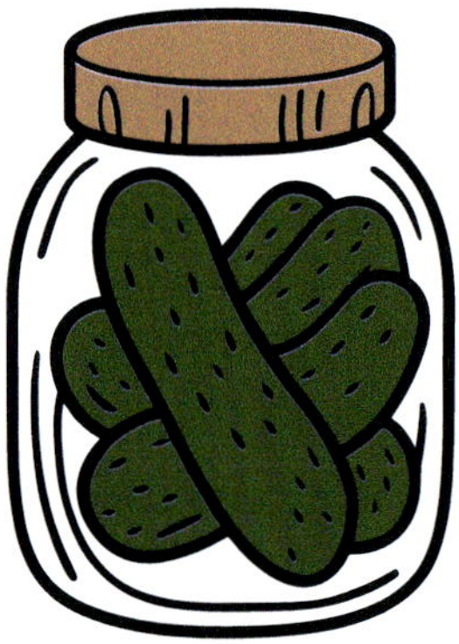

Menopause

Menopause can cause hormonal fluctuations, which can lead to: anxiety, brain fog, heart palpitations, hot flushes, weak bones, headaches, muscle and joint pain, a reduced sex drive, and many other symptoms.

Women who are menopausal are also at greater risk of developing type 2 diabetes because those hormonal fluctuations can lead to insulin resistance.

According to current research, altering one's lifestyle and adopting healthier behaviours, like those I have proposed in this book, can help to reduce hormone fluctuations, and improve insulin sensitivity.

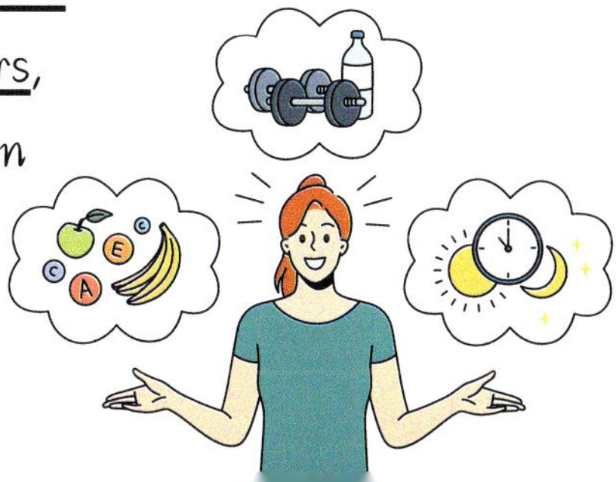

Dealing with menopause 149

It is generally recommended that women going through menopause should get adequate rest, exercise often, eat a balanced diet with plenty of calcium rich food, reduce their alcohol intake, and reduce or stop smoking.

I personally recommend making manageable changes that work for you. For example, if you are trying to exercise more but you have achy joints - swimming, water aerobics, or even just wading through the water can help. This is a great way of increasing your activity levels, while alleviating the pressure on your joints.

I would also recommend speaking with your GP about hormone replacement therapy and non-hormonal medications (which can help with night sweats and hot flushes).

Calcium rich foods:

- Dairy products
- Broccoli
- Cabbage
- Soya beans
- Tofu
- Almonds
- Brazil nuts
- Walnuts

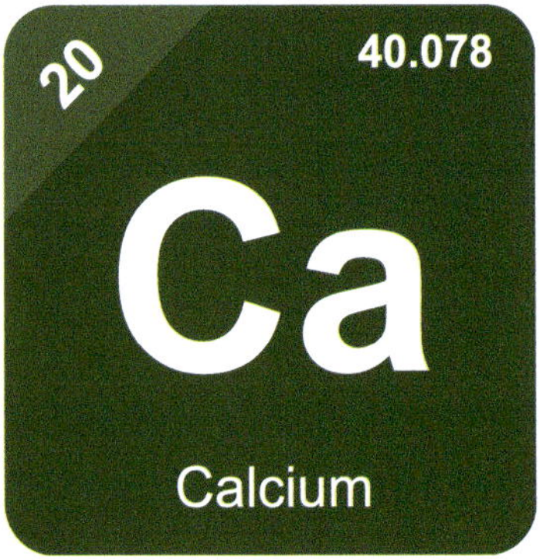

Polycystic ovary syndrome 150

Polycystic ovary syndrome, or PCOS, is the most common hormone related condition among women. Around 8-13% of women in the reproductive age have PCOS, and many are undiagnosed. It occurs when a woman develops cysts on her ovaries, preventing them from working correctly.

PCOS causes hormonal imbalances which can result in irregular menstruation, infertility, high blood pressure, high cholesterol, cardiovascular disease, endometrial cancer, obesity, depression, anxiety, excessive hair growth, thinning hair, acne, sleep apnoea, and type 2 diabetes.

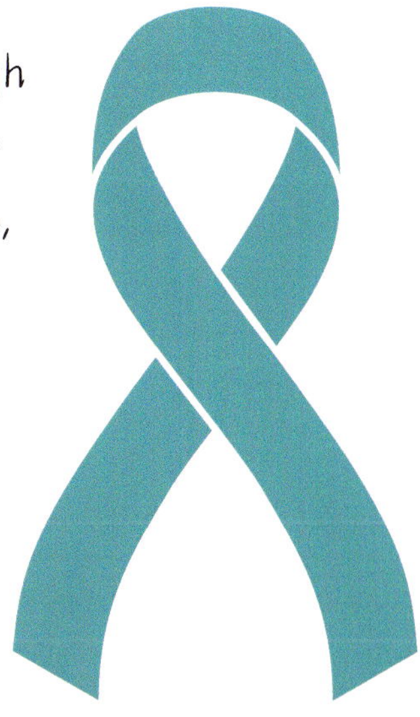

Unfortunately, PCOS cannot be cured, but the negative effects can be managed, as can your risk of developing type 2 diabetes.

Polycystic ovary syndrome

Lifestyle interventions are typically recommended for women with PCOS because they can help improve hormonal imbalances. The suggestions made throughout this book can help you to improve your diet, increase your activity levels, reduce your stress levels, improve sleep quality, and manage your weight, all of which can improve your experience of having PCOS.

However, if you are having issues with fertility, hair growth, hair loss, irregular menstruation, or you have any concerns, please do consult your GP.

Some women with PCOS do not develop symptoms, it is therefore important to have a pelvic exam and blood test in order to make sure and seek treatment if necessary.

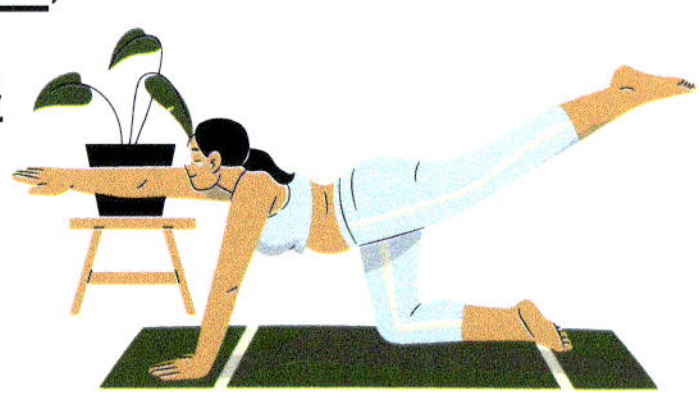

Cardiovascular disease

Any condition which affects the heart and blood vessels is considered a cardiovascular disease (CVD). There are currently 7.6 million people in the UK with some form of CVD, which causes around 25% of all deaths globally.

Cardiovascular disease is a common complication of type 2 diabetes, and affects around 32.2% of all diabetics.

Constant high blood sugar can cause bodily cells and nerves to deteriorate (page 14), resulting in your blood vessels being damaged. In turn, plaque begins to build up in those damaged areas and causes blockages and clots, potentially causing: angina, heart attacks, and strokes. This is how type 2 diabetes can lead to CVD.

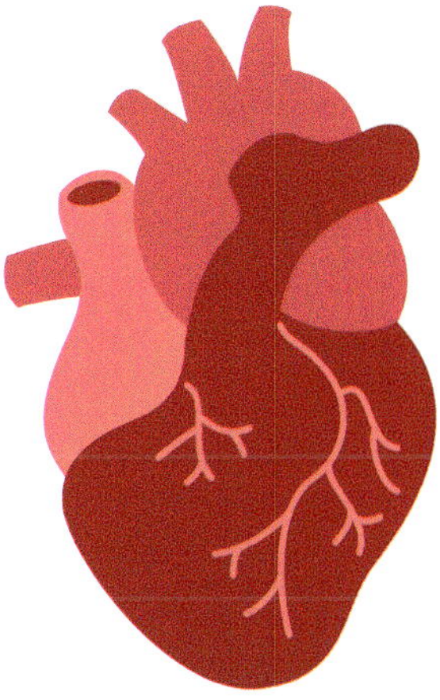

Overall, there is a lot of cross over between type 2 diabetes and cardiovascular disease - hence why it has been mentioned so frequently.

Cardiovascular disease can be caused by: your intake of fats, excessive amounts of salt, processed food, low levels of physical activity, stress, poor sleep, smoking, alcohol, inflammation, gut health, and more. There are also similar uncontrollable factors, such as: ethnicity, age, genetics, and PCOS.

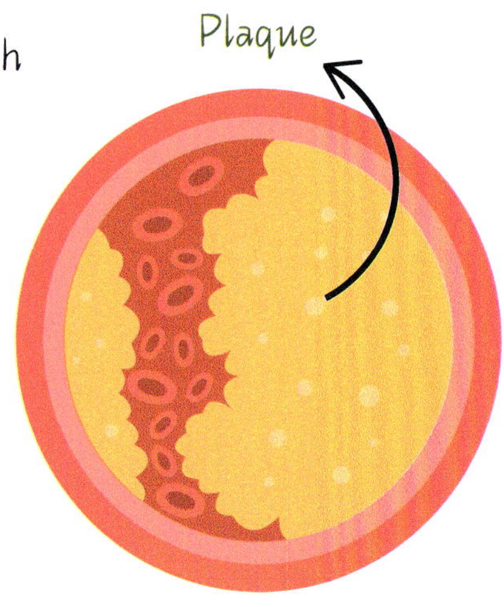

All of these factors have been explained in this guide. Therefore, if you follow the guidance, you will hopefully reduce your risk of developing type 2 diabetes and cardiovascular disease.

Depression

Depression is characterised by a generally negative outlook, and persistent feelings of sadness. It can last for long and short periods throughout a person's life, and can be a recurring problem. Medication is a solution for some people, but it isn't a route which works for everyone.

People often don't even recognise that they are depressed.

Symptoms of depression include;

- Struggling to concentrate
- Feeling excessive guilt
- A lack of self-worth
- A negative outlook on the future
- Poor sleep and insomnia
- Fluctuations in appetite or weight
- Feeling lethargic and fatigued
- Suicidal thoughts (in extreme cases)

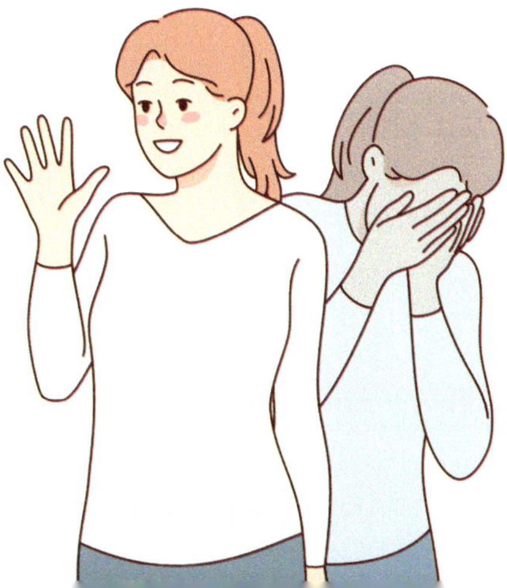

Depression and diabetes

People dealing with depression are more likely to be diagnosed with type 2 diabetes. Additionally, people with type 2 diabetes are more likely to develop depression. This, in part, is because many of the causes of type 2 diabetes also cause depression.

Depression can be caused by a poor diet, a lack of physical activity, stress, negative thoughts, a poor self image, family history, medication, a lack of sleep, hormonal changes, alcohol, drugs, inflammation, poor gut health, and more.

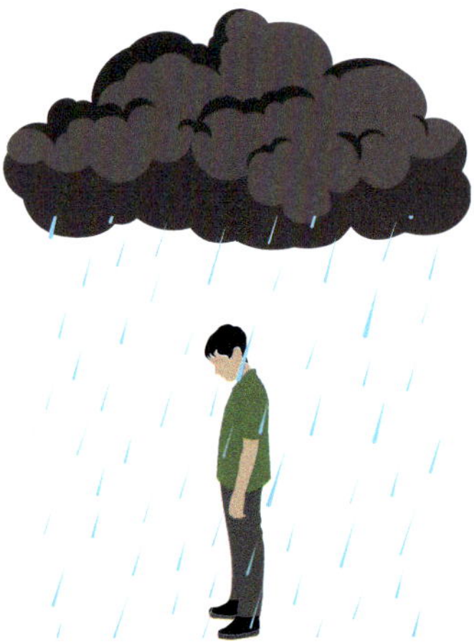

All of these factors have been addressed in this guide, and therefore, any changes you make with the intention of improving your physical health, can improve your mental health too!

Depression and motivation

Depression makes people feel alone and isolated.

It also drains those people of their motivation and willpower, often preventing them from making the very changes that could help them feel better.

Fortunately, small changes make a big difference.

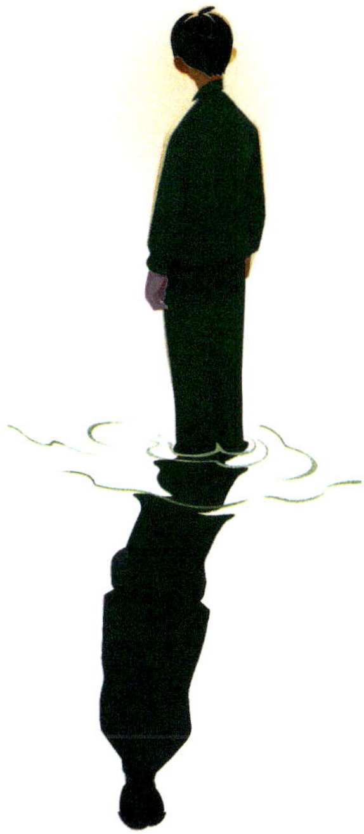

If you are dealing with depression, I hope this book has highlighted small changes you could see yourself making, and I truly hope you find that motivation. Just a short walk, or a chat with a friend can make a difference.

The final section is all about moving forward in a positive way, I would suggest using the tools and advice to make a plan for your future.

Reflection point 6

This is a list of suggestions based on the information from this section:

- Include anti-inflammatory foods in your diet to reduce your levels of inflammation.
- Include more prebiotic and probiotic foods in your diet to improve your gut health.
- Take a holistic approach to improving your health. Inflammation, oxidative stress, gut health, menopause, polycystic ovary syndrome, cardiovascular disease and depression all connect to type 2 diabetes in one way or another.
- Use this guide to reduce your risk of type 2 diabetes, in a manageable way. Doing so can also reduce the risk and severity of the conditions listed in this section!

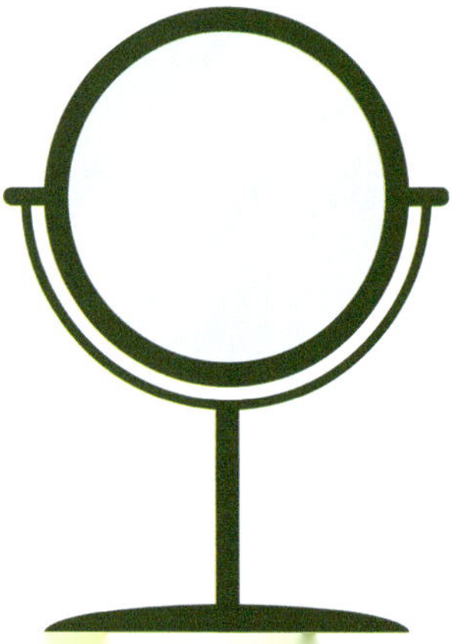

Section 7
MOVING FORWARD

"You should take care of, help, and
be good to yourself the same way you
would take care of, help, and be good
to someone you loved and valued."

— Jordan Peterson

Where do I start?

Improving your health can seem like an intimidating task, especially if you feel like the odds are stacked against you, and your health issues have begun to snowball in a negative direction.

That is why I believe it is important to weigh up the factors which you can and cannot control. For example, you cannot control your genetics, family history, medical history, age, or ethnicity.

Yet, this book demonstrates that there are many changes you can make, that are within your control. Where is the easiest place you can start? With just a few changes you can begin to snowball in a much more positive direction.

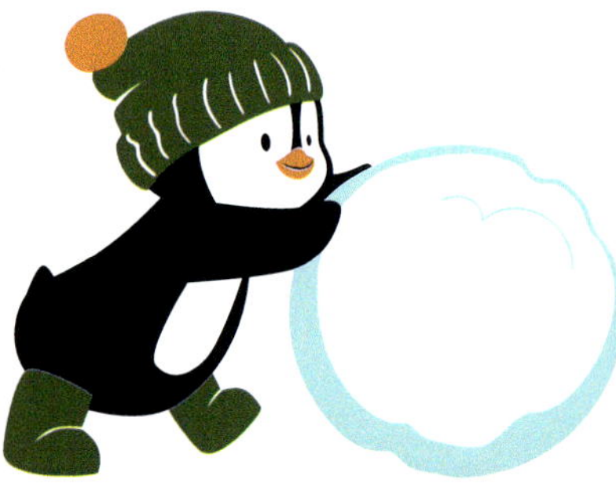

Balance and routine

The best advice I can give is to pick a topic from this book which resonates with you most and start by adding balance and routine to your daily and weekly habits.

You could start by adding balance to your intake of lower GI vs higher GI foods, activity vs inactivity, work vs rest, or any other aspect of your life which is tipped in a direction that is unhelpful for your general health, now and in the future.

You could also add healthy routines to your day to day, such as walking from a further bus stop, reading the food labels on meal-deals at lunch, and practicing breathing exercises to improve your stress levels and ability to fall asleep.

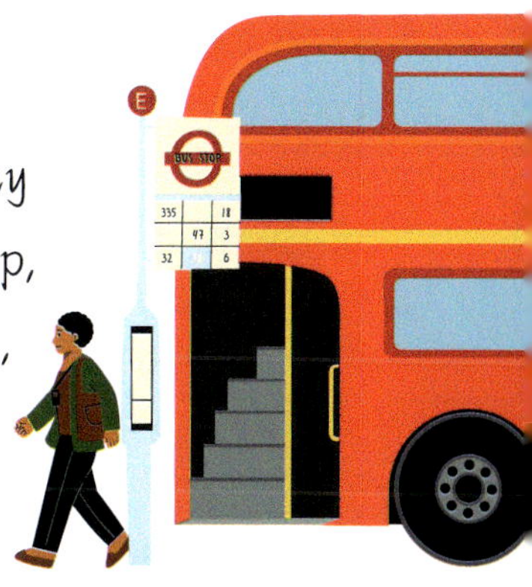

What is your aim?

Making a change without an aim is like going on a journey without a destination. To take the next steps, you must first know where you are going. You can then work backwards to understand the steps you need to take to make that happen!

To create your own aim, or set of aims, turn back to page 21 and answer the questions.

Here are a few example aims to inspire you:

- "I want to reduce my risk of type 2 diabetes"
- "I want to have more energy"
- "I want to live a longer and happier life"
- "I want to know how to improve my health"

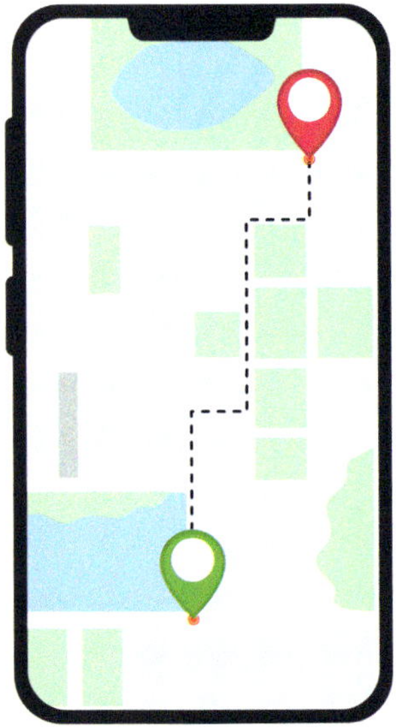

Once you have established your aim, you can use the next few pages to turn it into a plan. Start small, and don't tackle it all at once.

Making a plan

Below is an example of funnelling. As you progress down the table, the aim is broken down into a more manageable series of goals and actions. If you can then focus on your weekly and daily actions, the long term change will hopefully follow. This can be adapted to any aim, and can be reassessed and changed over time.

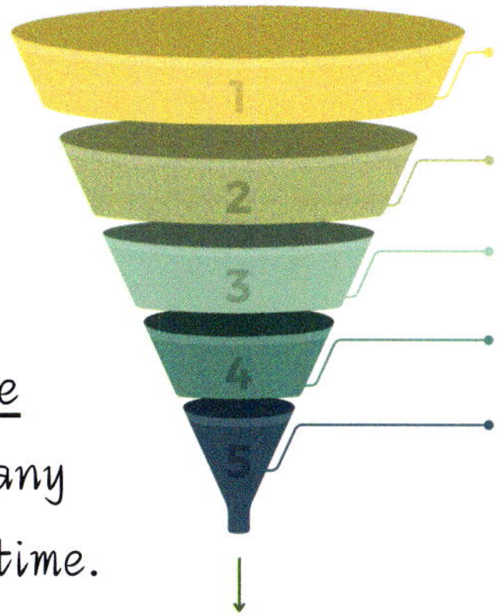

Aim	Reduce my risk of developing type 2 diabetes
Broad goal	Attempt to lose 10 pounds in 10 weeks
Specific goal	Attempt to lose 1 pound per week
Weekly actions	Go to a fitness class and swim once a week
Daily actions	Have wholegrain porridge and berries for breakfast

Expanded example

This is another example which has been expanded and is more specific.

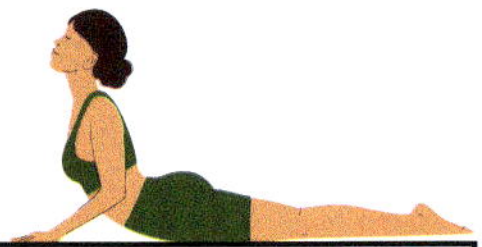

Aim	My aim is to reduce my risk of developing type 2 diabetes and stop feeling so anxious
Broad goal	Create a stress management plan which involves exercise and eating healthier comfort foods
Specific goal	Join a yoga class, learn breathing exercises, and begin reading food labels to find healthier comfort foods
Weekly actions	I could join a local yoga class every Thursday where they teach breathing exercises, and bring my friend
Daily actions	I could read the food labels to pick healthier snacks when I'm stressed at work

Try it yourself!

Answer the questions below to create your plan, and remember - there is no wrong way to do this!

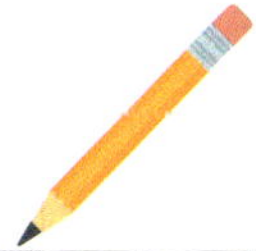

Aim	What is an aim that would give you direction, motivation, and purpose?
Broad goal	Based on the information from this guide, what is a broad goal that could help you work towards your aim?
Specific goal	Can you break this down into a more manageable and specific goal, or series of goals?
Weekly actions	Based on the information from this guide, what actions could you take this week to achieve your goals?
Daily actions	Based on the information from this guide, what actions could you take today to achieve your goals?

Navigating the map

As I said at the beginning of the book, and as I have demonstrated throughout - health is like a complex map that has many routes, and improving your health is a journey!

A practical approach is best.

Zoom out, consider all of factors which affect your health, use the information in this book to find the route which will work for you, and make a plan! If you ever find yourself lost, don't beat yourself up, reassess and continue.

Success is in the efforts.

Good luck! I hope you reach your destination, and that you enjoy the journey.

Can you find me on the front cover?

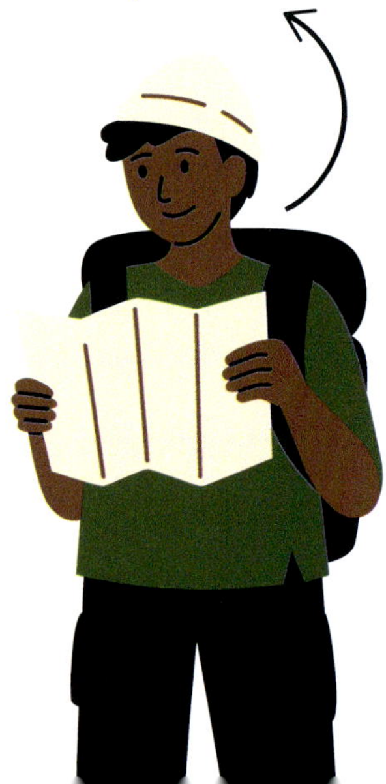

Thank you for reading!

I'm incredibly thankful to everybody who purchased this book, read it, and shared it. I have poured my heart into researching, writing, and designing it for almost 2 years and I have learnt so much in the process.

My aim was to make a resource that would help people. I genuinely hope that this book has given you something, be it information, motivation, or just food for thought. My hope is that you will keep this book close by, refer back to it whenever you need assistance, and that you will use it to teach your children to take care of their health as well. On the final pages are a number of links, references, and my contact details. Feel free to reach out if you have any questions or feedback.

I wish you good health!

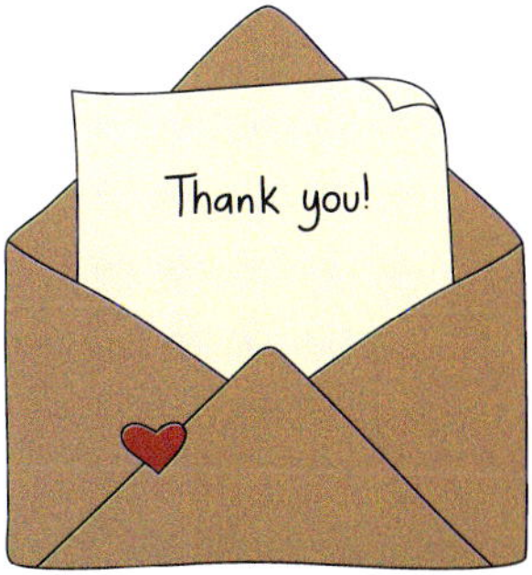

Keep in touch!

I love answering questions, so please get in touch if you have <u>any</u> questions at all. If you would like to attend my Health Support programme, or any of my upcoming events, the details will be on my website. I also run health seminars and workshops for businesses and charities.

Here is how you can reach me...

My Instagram:
@zacharymartinpt

My website:
www.zmpt-health.com

My email address:
zachary.martin@zmpt-health.com

Health Support

'Health Support' is a community programme which I deliver in London and Essex. I teach about a range of topics, including: nutrition, stress, sleep, physical activity, inflammation, gut health, weight, addiction, type 2 diabetes, cardiovascular disease, blood pressure, cholesterol, and much more.

If you would like to attend these sessions, please visit my website or get in touch using the details on the previous page.

Anyone and everyone is welcome, and sessions are taking place every month. Feel free to come along if you ever need support, and send an invite to someone who would benefit!

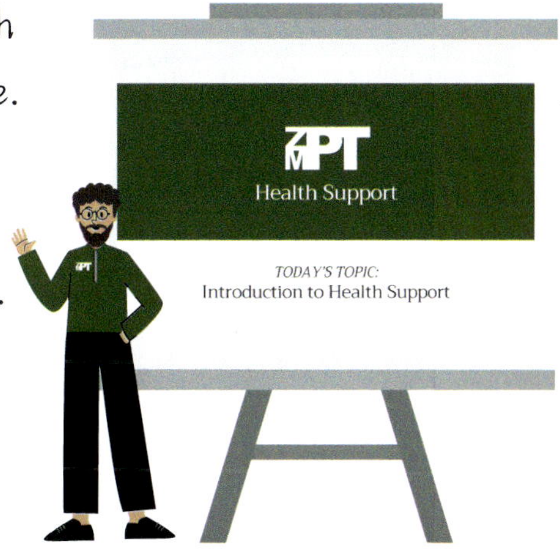

Diabetes UK local support groups
(www.diabetes.org.uk/support-for-you/community-support-and-forums/local-support-groups)

NHS Diabetes Prevention Programme
(www.england.nhs.uk/diabetes/diabetes-prevention)

NHS mental health services
(www.nhs.uk/nhs-services/mental-health-services)

NHS Live Well page
(www.nhs.uk/live-well)

NHS smoking support
(www.nhs.uk/live-well/quit-smoking/nhs-stop-smoking-services-help-you-quit)

Sane
(www.sane.org.uk)

Samaritans
(www.samaritans.org)

Drink aware
(www.drinkaware.co.uk/advice-and-support/alcohol-support-services)

Age UK physical activity support
(www.ageuk.org.uk/services/in-your-area/exercise)

Nuffield joint pain programme
(www.nuffieldhealth.com/about-us/our-impact/healthy-life/joint-pain-programme)

Glycemic index guide
(www.glycemicindex.com)

- NHS, Diabetes
(www.nhs.uk/conditions/diabetes/)

- NHS, Stress
(www.nhs.uk/mental-health/conditions/post-traumatic-stress-disorder-ptsd/overview/)

- NHS, PTSD
(www.nhs.uk/mental-health/conditions/post-traumatic-stress-disorder-ptsd/overview/)

- NHS, Anxiety
(www.nhs.uk/mentalhealth/conditions/generalised-anxiety-disorder-gad/)

- NHS, Polycystic ovary syndrome
(www.nhs.uk/mental-health/conditions/post-traumatic-stress-disorder-ptsd/overview/)

- NHS, Depression
(www.nhs.uk/mentalhealth/conditions/depression-in-adults/overview/)

- NHS, Sweeteners
(www.nhs.uk/live-well/eat-well/food-types/are-sweeteners-safe/)

- NHS, Vaping
(www.nhs.uk/better-health/quit-smoking/ready-to-quit-smoking/vaping-to-quit-smoking/vaping-myths-and-the-facts/)

- NHS, Menopause
(www.nhs.uk/conditions/menopause/)

- NHS, Coronary heart disease
(www.nhs.uk/conditions/coronary-heart-disease/)

- WHO, Tobacco
(www.who.int/news-room/fact-sheets/detail/tobacco)

- WHO, Healthy diet
(www.who.int/news-room/fact-sheets/detail/healthy-diet)

- WHO, Cardiovascular diseases (www.who.int/news-room/fact sheets/detail/cardiovascular-diseases-(cvds)

- WHO, Sweeteners (www.who.int/news/item/15-05-2023-who-advises-not-to-use-non-sugar-sweeteners-for-weight-control-in-newly-released-guideline)

- WHO, Menopause (www.who.int/news-room/fact-sheets/detail/menopause)

- WHO, Physical activity (www.who.int/news-room/fact-sheets/detail/physical-activity)

- WHO, Polycystic Ovary Syndrome (www.who.int/news-room/fact-sheets/detail/polycystic-ovary-syndrome)

- WHO, Depression (www.who.int/news-room/fact-sheets/detail/depression)

- WHO, Mental health (www.who.int/news-room/fact-sheets/detail/mental-health-strengthening-our-response)

- WHO, Sodium (www.who.int/news-room/fact-sheets/detail/sodium-reduction)

- WHO, Trans fats (www.who.int/news-room/fact-sheets/detail/trans-fat)

- WHO, Ageing and health (www.who.int/news-room/fact-sheets/detail/ageing-and-health)

- Adams, O. P. (2013). The impact of brief high-intensity exercise on blood glucose levels.
- Advisory, S. (2003). Salt and Health.
- Ahmed, A. U. (2011). An overview of inflammation: mechanism and consequences.
- Al-Ishaq, R. K., et al. (2019). Flavonoids and their anti-diabetic effects.
- Alberts, B., et al. (2002). How cells obtain energy from food.
- Anderson, J. W., Baird, P., Davis Jr, R. H., Ferreri, S., Knudtson, M., Koraym, A., ... & Williams, C. L. (2009). Health benefits of dietary fiber.
- Aslam, H., et al. (2020). Fermented foods, the gut and mental health.
- Atkinson, F. S., Brand-Miller, J. C., Foster-Powell, K., Buyken, A. E., & Goletzke, J. (2021). International tables of glycemic index and glycemic load values 2021: a systematic review.
- Awuchi, C. G., & Echeta, K. C. (2019). Current developments in sugar alcohols.
- Bahman, M., et al. (2018). The importance of sleep hygiene in polycystic ovary syndrome.
- Barber, T. M., & Franks, S. (2021). Obesity and polycystic ovary syndrome.
- Berryman, J. W. (2012). Motion and rest: Galen on exercise and health.
- Bhattacharya, P., et al. (2023). Impact of exercise on brain neurochemicals.
- Brimson, J. M., et al. (2021). Role of herbal teas in regulating cellular homeostasis.
- Burger, H. G., et al. (2002). Hormonal changes in the menopause transition.
- Cabib, S., & Puglisi-Allegra, S. (2012). The mesoaccumbens dopamine in coping with stress.
- Cannon, W. B. (1929). Organization for physiological homeostasis.
- Carlsen, M. H., Halvorsen, B. L., Holte, K., Bohn, S. K., Dragland, S., Rossland, L. M., ... Blomhoff, R. (2010). The total antioxidant content of more than 3100 foods, beverages, spices, herbs and supplements used worldwide.

- Childs, E., & de Wit, H. (2009). Hormonal, cardiovascular, and subjective responses to acute stress in smokers.
- Clauss, M., et al. (2021). Interplay between exercise and gut microbiome.
- Darwish, L., et al. (2018). Depression in people with type 2 diabetes.
- Daubenmier, J. J., et al. (2007). The contribution of changes in diet, exercise, and stress management.
- De Heredia, F. P., et al. (2012). Obesity, inflammation and the immune system.
- Dhaka, V., Gulia, N., Ahlawat, K. S., & Khatkar, B. S. (2011). Trans fats—sources, health risks and alternative approach - a review.
- Dhingra, D., Michael, M., Rajput, H., & Patil, R. T. (2012). Dietary fibre in foods: a review.
- Dutta, M., Das, P., & Bhattacharyaa, S. (2025). Understanding prebiotics: A review on their role, benefits, and applications.
- Einarson, T. R., et al. (2018). Prevalence of cardiovascular disease in type 2 diabetes.
- Eliasson, B. R., et al. (1996). Long-term use of nicotine gum.
- Emanuele, N. V., et al. (1998). Consequences of alcohol use in diabetics.
- Fan, Y., & Pedersen, O. (2021). Gut microbiota in human metabolic health and disease.
- Fathallah, N., et al. (2015). Drug-induced hyperglycaemia and diabetes.
- Feingold, K. R. (2024). Introduction to lipids and lipoproteins.
- Foster, J. A., et al. (2017). Stress & the gut-brain axis.
- Foster-Powell, K., & Miller, J. B. (1995). International tables of glycemic index.
- Goldstein, J. L., & Brown, M. S. (2009). The LDL receptor.
- Guilliams, T. G., & Edwards, L. (2010). Chronic stress and the HPA axis.
- Gurung, M., et al. (2020). Role of gut microbiota in type 2 diabetes pathophysiology.

- Hadlow, N. C., Brown, S., Wardrop, R., & Henley, D. (2014). The effects of season, daylight saving and time of sunrise on serum cortisol in a large population.
- Hartley, T. R., Lovallo, W. R., Whitsett, T. L., Sung, B. H., & Wilson, M. F. (2001). Caffeine and stress: implications for risk, assessment, and management of hypertension.
- Hantsoo, L., & Zemel, B. S. (2021). Stress gets into the belly.
- Imai, S., et al. (2014). Effect of eating vegetables before carbohydrates.
- Imamura, F., Micha, R., Wu, J. H., de Oliveira Otto, M. C., Otite, F. O., Abioye, A. I., & Mozaffarian, D. (2016). Effects of saturated fat, polyunsaturated fat, monounsaturated fat, and carbohydrate on glucose-insulin homeostasis: a systematic review and meta-analysis of randomised controlled feeding trials.
- Jaehne, A., et al. (2009). Effects of nicotine on sleep during consumption, withdrawal and replacement therapy.
- Bahman, M., et al. (2018). The importance of sleep hygiene in polycystic ovary syndrome.
- Barber, T. M., & Franks, S. (2021). Obesity and polycystic ovary syndrome.
- Berryman, J. W. (2012). Motion and rest: Galen on exercise and health.
- Bhattacharya, P., et al. (2023). Impact of exercise on brain neurochemicals.
- Brimson, J. M., et al. (2021). Role of herbal teas in regulating cellular homeostasis.
- Burger, H. G., et al. (2002). Hormonal changes in the menopause transition.
- Cabib, S., & Puglisi-Allegra, S. (2012). The mesoaccumbens dopamine in coping with stress.
- Cannon, W. B. (1929). Organization for physiological homeostasis.
- Carlsen, M. H., Halvorsen, B. L., Holte, K., Bohn, S. K., Dragland, S., Rossland, L. M., ... Blomhoff, R. (2010). The total antioxidant content of more than 3100 foods, beverages, spices, herbs and supplements used worldwide.

- LeMoult, J., & Gotlib, I. H. (2019). Depression: A cognitive perspective.
- Lenhart, A., & Chey, W. D. (2017). A systematic review of the effects of polyols
- Li, C. J., et al. (2015). Effects of a macro-nutrient preload.
- Liu, A. G., Ford, N. A., Hu, F. B., Zelman, K. M., Mozaffarian, D., & Kris-Etherton, P. M. (2017). A healthy approach to dietary fats: understanding the science and taking action to reduce consumer confusion.
- Lovallo, W. R., et al. (2006). Cortisol responses to mental stress.
- Lu, C. C., & Yen, G. C. (2015). Antioxidative and anti-inflammatory activity.
- Lukaschek, K., et al. (2013). Relationship between posttraumatic stress disorder and Type 2 Diabetes.
- Mailing, L. J., et al. (2019). Exercise and the gut microbiome.
- Marco, M. L., Sanders, M. E., Gänzle, M., Arrieta, M. C., Cotter, P. D., De Vuyst, L., ... & Hutkins, R. (2021). The International Scientific Association for Probiotics and Prebiotics (ISAPP) consensus statement on fermented foods.
- Mason, I. C., et al. (2020). Impact of circadian disruption on glucose metabolism.
- Metsios, G. S., et al. (2020). Exercise and inflammation.
- Mikkelsen, K., et al. (2017). Exercise and mental health.
- Mogol, B. A., & Gökmen, V. (2016). Thermal process contaminants: Acrylamide, chloropropanols and furan.
- Monteiro, C. A., et al. (2019). Ultra-processed foods.
- National Research Council. (1989). Diet and health: Implications for reducing chronic disease risk.

- Nayak, P. K., Dash, U. M. A., Rayaguru, K., & Krishnan, K. R. (2016). Physio-chemical changes during repeated frying of cooked oil: A Review.
- Neal, D. T., et al. (2006). Habits—A repeat performance.
- Pagliai, G., et al. (2021). Consumption of ultra-processed foods.
- Pal, G. K., & Velkumary, S. (2004). Effect of short-term practice of breathing exercises.
- Patel, A. K., Reddy, V., Shumway, K. R., & Araujo, J. F. (2024). Physiology, sleep stages
- Patterson, M. S., et al. (2022). Exercise in the treatment of addiction.
- Peteliuk, V., et al. (2021). Natural sweetener Stevia rebaudiana.
- Petersen, K. S., Maki, K. C., Calder, P. C., Belury, M. A., Messina, M., Kirkpatrick, C. F., & Harris, W. S. (2024). Perspective on the health effects of unsaturated fatty acids and commonly consumed plant oils high in unsaturated fat.
- Reith, C., et al. (2024). Effects of statin therapy.
- Rezvani, A. H., & Levin, E. D. (2001). Cognitive effects of nicotine.
- Roberts, A. L., et al. (2015). Posttraumatic stress disorder and type 2 diabetes.
- Rohm, T. V., et al. (2022). Inflammation in obesity, diabetes, and related disorders.
- Saad, A., et al. (2014). A Review on potential toxicity of artificial sweetners.
- Sahi, A., et al. (1985). Modulation of glycemic response.
- Schilström, B., et al. (2003). Dual effects of nicotine on dopamine neurons.
- Selye, H. (1950). Stress and the general adaptation syndrome.
- Simpson, N., & Dinges, D. F. (2007). Sleep and inflammation.
- Singh, S. D., & Rao, G. P. (2005). Stevia: The herbal sugar of 21st century.

- Slopien, R., et al. (2018). Menopause and diabetes.
- Snel, J., & Lorist, M. M. (2011). Effects of caffeine on sleep and cognition.
- Sonia, S., et al. (2015). Effect of cooling of cooked white rice.
- Spencer, R. L., & Hutchison, K. E. (1999). Alcohol, aging, and the stress response.
- Su, Q., & Liu, Q. (2021). Factors affecting gut microbiome in daily diet.
- Tipton, C. M. (2014). The history of "Exercise Is Medicine".
- Tristan Asensi, M., et al. (2023). Low-grade inflammation and ultra-processed foods.
- Wang, M., & Hng, T. M. (2021). HbA1c: More than just a number.
- Wee, M. S., & Henry, C. J. (2020). Reducing the glycemic impact of carbohydrates.
- Wilcox, G. (2005). Insulin and insulin resistance.
- Wise, R. A., & Robble, M. A. (2020). Dopamine and addiction.
- Wronka, M., Krzemińska, J., Młynarska, E., Rysz, J., & Franczyk, B. (2022). The influence of lifestyle and treatment on oxidative stress and inflammation in diabetes.
- Xie, X. T., et al. (2009). Impact of cigarette smoking in type 2 diabetes.
- Yan, L., et al. (2022). Physical exercise prevented stress-induced anxiety.
- Yu, X., Pu, H., & Voss, M. (2024). Overview of anti-inflammatory diets and their promising effects on non-communicable diseases.
- Zunszain, P. A., et al. (2013). Inflammation and depression.

- Brian Luke Seaward. (2006). Managing stress: principles and strategies for health and wellbeing.
- British Heart Foundation. (2025). British Heart Foundation, UK Factsheet.
- Cannon, W. B. (1915). Bodily changes in pain, hunger, fear and rage: An account of recent researches into the function of emotional excitement.
- Healthy eating habits 2 for patients with diabetes - A noncommunicable disease education manual for primary health care professionals and patients. (2015). World Health Organisation.
- Mcardle, W. D., Katch, F. I., & Katch, V. L. (2016). Essentials of exercise physiology (5th ed.).
- NHS England. (2022). Children and young people with diabetes: An interactive toolkit for healthcare professionals.
- Parker, S. (2019). The concise human body book.
- Porter, R. (2001). The Cambridge illustrated history of medicine. Cambridge University Press.
- Shook, S. (2022). The Science of Sleep. Kapi'olani Community College.
- Souter, K. (2015). Your Guide to Understanding and Dealing with Type 2 Diabetes.
- Sproule, J. (2012). Sports, exercise and health science course companion. Oxford University Press.
- WHO guidelines on physical activity and sedentary behaviour. (2020). World Health Organisation.

The blurb

This is a guide through the world of health and how it relates to TYPE 2 DIABETES.

TYPE 2 DIABETES is a complex topic that is often misunderstood. There are many factors which determine whether you develop it - it is not just sugary food! Factors such as general nutrition, physical activity, chronic stress, lack of sleep, inflammation, and much more!

I made this book for 3 reasons.
Health can be boring.
Health can be nuanced.
Health can be confusing.

That is why this book is easy to understand, and styled like a fun children's book.

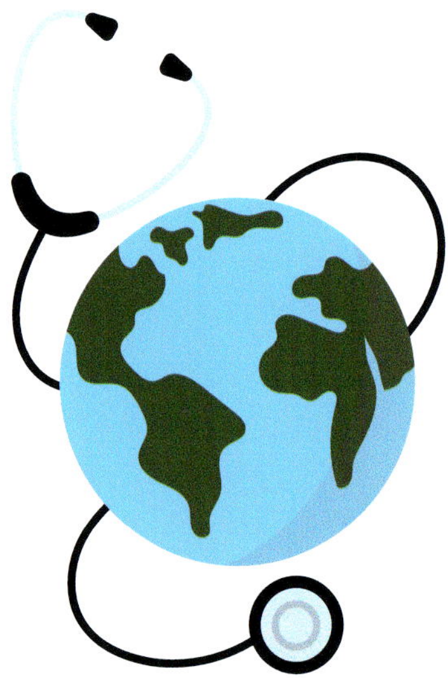

* 9 7 8 1 9 1 9 2 8 3 3 0 2 *

BV - #0055 - 030226 - C187 - 152/152/13 - PB - 9781919283302 - Gloss Lamination